The Complete

Diabetes Organizer

Your Guide to a Less Stressful and More Manageable Diabetes Life

SUSAN WEINER and LESLIE JOSEL

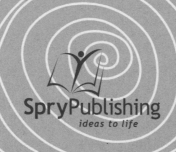

SpryPublishing
ideas to life

This edition is published by Spry Publishing LLC

2500 South State Street

Ann Arbor, MI 48104 USA

Printed and bound in China.

10   9   8   7   6   5   4   3   2   1

Library of Congress Control Number: 2013937937

Paperback ISBN: 978-1-938170-26-3

E-book ISBN: 978-1-938170-27-0

App lists included in this book are adapted from *An App a Day* and *An App a Day for Health Professionals*, © 2012, Frederico Arts LLC.

App lists included in this book are not intended to be complete lists and represent only a sample of apps available on the topics. New apps will become available over time. These app lists are for informational purposes only and make no endorsements or claims about the quality of the apps. Frederico Arts LLC is not responsible for app availability, content, function, reliability, or use outcomes. App price, content, and availability are subject to change. Please consult your personal doctor and medical team for advice that pertains to your specific individual needs.

Disclaimer: Spry Publishing LLC does not assume responsibility for the contents or opinions expressed herein. Although every precaution is taken to ensure that information is accurate as of the date of publication, differences of opinion exist. The opinions expressed herein are those of the authors and do not necessarily reflect the views of the publisher. The information contained in this book is not intended to replace professional advisement of an individual's doctor prior to beginning or changing an individual's course of treatment.

To Ed, Ben, and Steven for their support and encouragement.
Also to the loving memory of my father, Harold Greenberg, whose
wisdom and honesty continue to guide me. A special dedication
to my patients and the entire diabetes community—
may you be blessed with good health and a cure.

—SW

To my husband, Wayne, my true partner in every way.
And to Maddie and Eli who allow me to hone my organizing
skills every day. And a special dedication to my dear
friends Liza and Michael, who in my book are the true heroes.

—LJ

A portion of the author's royalties have been donated to the
Diabetes Hands Foundation www.diabeteshandsfoundation.org

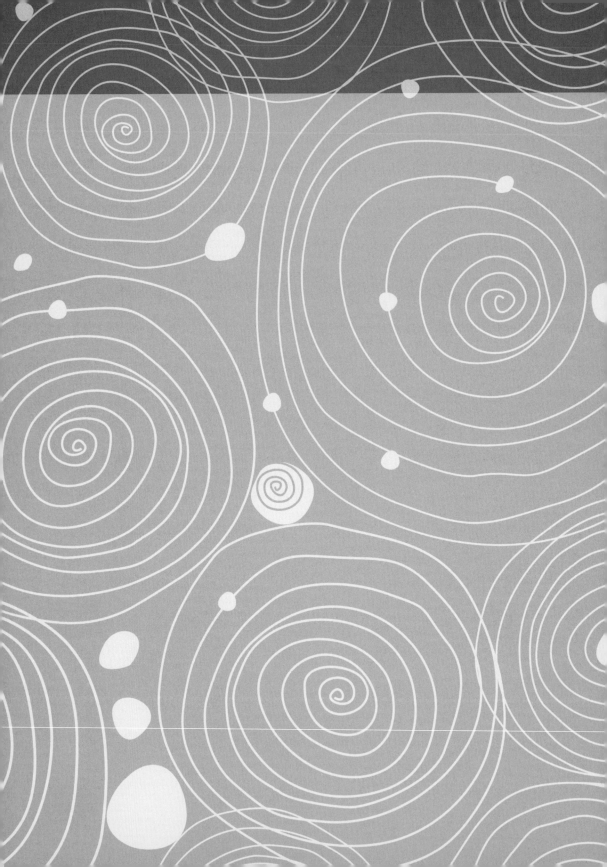

Contents

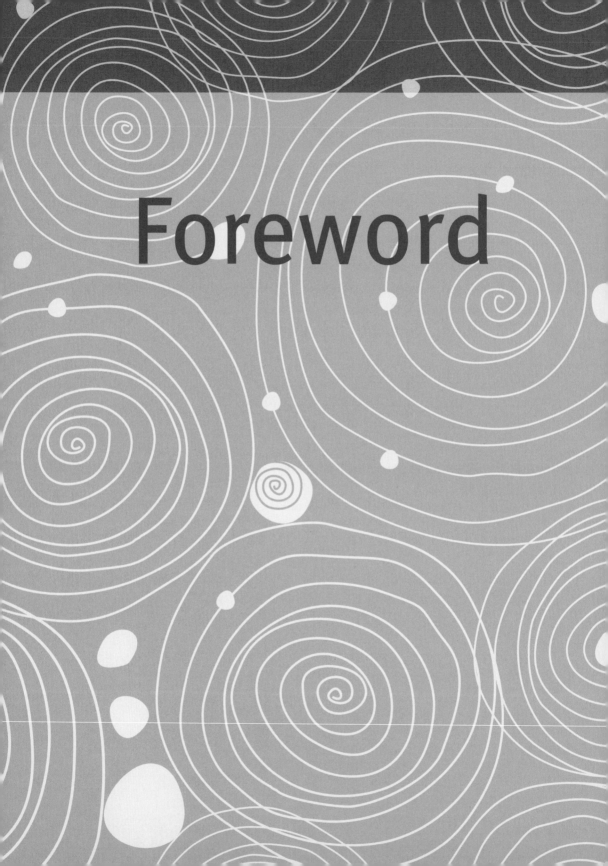

Foreword

DIABETES HAS BEEN DECLARED to be the fastest growing epidemic in history. Yet, for many, diabetes is a mystery. Those who don't live with diabetes or live with someone with diabetes are often surprised to learn just how devastating diabetes can be. They don't understand why so many people must lose their lives, their vision, or their kidneys or limbs to diabetes. They wonder why such horrible consequences occur or why people with diabetes don't take better care of themselves if the consequences of poorly managed diabetes can be so dire.

The answer is simple. Diabetes is complex and diabetes is HARD. It's not just about simply avoiding sugar or taking medication or insulin. It requires doing for yourself what your body would ordinarily do for you. You must learn new things, sometimes complex new things, and adopt a whole new set of daily behaviors and dietary restrictions. And it's not just about being better informed. It takes motivation, persistence, and *organization* to be a "successful" diabetes patient. It's hard and it never takes a day off. Never. But with all that said, I've managed to keep this monster under control for more than 43 years and lead a very active personal and professional life.

No one chooses to have diabetes. It chooses you. And if it chooses you and if you're like me, not the most organized person, it makes managing the daily grind of diabetes that much harder. Getting up and getting to work or school on time, having the right food with you, leaving enough time to test your blood sugar, finding the right meal options, record keeping, traveling, and expecting the unexpected are all part of the game of diabetes management. The consequences of disorganization take on an intensely more serious dimension with diabetes than it might otherwise have in life.

That's why I love this book. It *makes* better diabetes organizers. Combining the expertise and experience of a compassionate and accomplished diabetes educator with a professional organizational expert provides an uncommon and highly practical approach—a potential game changer for those with busy schedules who want to get the most out of life while optimizing, not sacrificing, diabetes management. Finally, a realistic guide to accomplish all of your personal and professional goals as someone living with diabetes.

From the moment I wake up to the time I go to bed and even while asleep, my life must be organized for my diabetes health. I believe it was the legendary coach John Wooden who said, "Failure to plan is a plan to fail." That is the ultimate truism in diabetes. I organize my life so that diabetes doesn't slow me down and life doesn't overwhelm my diabetes, and this book can help you do the same. Forgetting supplies or eating the wrong thing because you are not organized for the diabetes day is what throws off the delicate balance of control. What I have with me for a dog walk or in the office, how I pack for a trip, it can matter a lot. And the better you plan and organize, the more peace of mind you have for yourself or for caring for someone else with diabetes—particularly true for parents of children with diabetes.

While there are many paths to good control, I'm not sure I would be here today, 43 years after I was diagnosed, in very good health, if not for organizing my life with diabetes as a priority. I would be of little value to my family, the community, colleagues, and myself if I didn't maintain that vigilance.

We all lead busy lives, made more complex and pressured by a chronic condition called diabetes, but what choice do we have but to do the best we can and take advantage of great tools like *The Complete Diabetes Organizer: Your Guide to a Less Stressful and More Manageable Diabetes Life?* Some days will be harder than others, but if you're reading this, you already took a big step toward getting your diabetes house in order. *Everyone* can use some help organizing their day, their week, and their life to better manage diabetes. This book connects all people with diabetes and addresses all aspects of diabetes to help you stay focused, organized, and in control.

It's your diabetes life. Own it!

Howard Steinberg, dLife Founder

Chapter One

Let's Get Organized!

HOW DID YOU FEEL when your diabetes was diagnosed or when you learned that your spouse or child had diabetes? Were you angry or scared? Were you bombarded with information from your doctor about diet, exercise, and lifestyle changes? How did you handle unwanted advice from family members and friends about managing your blood sugar? Did you ignore the diagnosis because you were already overwhelmed with your daily schedule and to-do lists? If so, you're not alone!

Hopefully, you already know that your diabetes doesn't define you, but your diabetes is part of you. And, you are challenged every day to organize your daily activities and diabetes care so that you can help prevent complications associated with diabetes. Heart disease, kidney disease, blindness, and stroke can all be the result of poorly managed diabetes. In this book, we'll offer strategies to help you organize your diabetes, manage your blood sugars, and improve your health. We are here to guide you every step of the way. So, let's do this together!

Getting Started

For those of you who may be newly diagnosed, we know you are feeling overwhelmed at this moment. Your life has taken an unexpected turn and you're on information overload. There are endless lists of medical information and "must-have" products and supplies for your diabetes. You've been told to put critical systems into place immediately. You might even feel as if you're ducking major-league curve balls from all directions.

The wheels are turning and the mental "to-do" list is running through your head. In fact, your list might look something like this:

- Make room for daily or weekly exercise.
- Pack my lunch for work every day.
- Test my blood 3 times a day while traveling for work.
- Organize necessary supplies and food.
- Communicate critical information to those around me—friends, coworkers, doctors, insurance representatives.

For those of you who have been dealing with diabetes for some time, those same challenges and to-do lists still apply. And, on top of those daily items, you may be experiencing burnout and the mental fatigue that come from managing the constant demands of diabetes care.

It's enough to make you want to pull the covers over your head and hide. We don't blame you. How do you make sense of it all? How do you make sure you get done what needs to get done? How do you fit it all in your already busy life? That's where we come in.

Where to Start

And, at the risk of over-simplifying things, the first step to improving your diabetes life is pretty basic—set your goals. Yes, you heard us. Set goals.

Now you may ask what do goals have to do with a diabetes diagnosis? Everything! If you take on too much and remain disorganized, your thoughts will scatter in a million directions. Your goals and priorities might remain unclear and confused. Your personal goals are crucial to helping you succeed in all areas of your life. Setting goals will prevent you from becoming overwhelmed and will improve your focus. In other words, goal setting will allow you to create the roadmap to get you to where you want to go.

> "*Setting goals has always been my way of yelling at myself. 'Jim! Pay attention!'* "
>
> JIM TURNER, actor and comedian, diagnosed at age 17 with type 1 diabetes

In order to reach any goal, you have to begin by defining it. Please don't skip this step. You'll find that it's a very important part of your journey toward better health and improved diabetes management. Since your situation is so unique, it is crucial to get a clear picture of where you are and where you are headed before you take another step forward. Use the questions on page 15 to gain some insight into your challenges and develop your individual goals.

Here's what your roadmap might look like:

1. **Look forward.** Ask yourself what you hope to accomplish. Where do you want to be? Envision the end result.

2. **Write goals.** Writing your goals will help you remember all that you want to achieve.

3. **Create an action plan.** Be realistic. It's much easier to accomplish a goal when it is broken down into manageable parts than trying to tackle it as a whole.

4. **Plan time.** Schedule appointments with yourself and set due dates. Having a deadline is motivating!

5. **Activate.** Be positive. If you believe you will accomplish it, you will do it.

6. **Recognize road blocks.** Plan for imperfection. You might get off track from time to time. Be kind to yourself.

7. **Set up supports.** Tell a friend. Ask for help. Buddy up. Sharing your plan with others can help you stay on task.

8. **Look back.** See where you've been. Take stock. Learn from both your accomplishments and your mistakes.

9. **Relish rewards.** Treat yourself along the way with small rewards to help stay motivated.

10. **Stay on track.** Keep your eye on the prize. Pace yourself. Remember, this is a marathon, not a sprint.

Considerations for Goal Setting

What aspects of diabetes management challenge you the most?

_____

_____

What needs to change in your household, life, or schedule?

_____

_____

What could you do to make those changes?

_____

_____

What strategies could you use to stick with those changes long-term?

_____

_____

Are there already certain systems in place that could help you achieve your goals?

_____

_____

Were you able to answer most or all of those questions? Start to identify what works and what needs to be changed or altered and you're on the path to defining your goals. Find some uninterrupted time (you may need to set time aside in your schedule to keep this "appointment"), a quiet spot, and take a deep breath. It is time to write down those goals!

Think SMART! Make your goals

Specific
Measurable
Actionable
Relevant
Timely

Setting Your Goals

In the space on page 18, record your diabetes organizational or management goals. In each case, consider the likelihood that you can achieve the goal you are setting. If you don't feel that you are "likely" or "very likely" to stick with the goal, consider revising it slightly to make it more likely that you will follow through. Don't bite off more than you can chew and you will be more likely to accomplish your goals.

Consider this: Were you setting a goal of exercising an hour every day? Goals should not be specific tasks. However, a goal can be accomplished by completing a task over a specific period of time. For example, let's say that the goal you set is to exercise more often. If you go to the gym on a Tuesday morning, that doesn't mean you have achieved your goal. (Although it is a great start!) You have completed a task toward your goal. If you go to the gym every Tuesday morning, you are on your way to achieving that goal. Don't get discouraged if you miss a Tuesday morning either! It doesn't mean you can't achieve your goal as long as you find an alternate time for your exercise.

Please remember that change is a process. Don't try to change everything at once. Pick one of your goals to work on at a time. Once you accomplish that goal, move on to the next one.

Create an Action Plan

So now you've defined your goals, but how do you start to achieve them? How long will it take to accomplish your goals? How are you going to get there? In order to answer these questions, you'll need to develop an action plan. Let's come up with a strategy that works for you.

Think about a strategy or action plan for a specific goal that you want to achieve. Do you have a system already in place that relates to that goal? Next, think about what you may be able to realistically adapt or change to achieve your newly defined goal. Identify and preserve what works for you. Many times, making a change doesn't require that you redo everything, especially if you already have systems in place that work somewhat for you. Perhaps your system only needs to be slightly tweaked.

> Jim Turner says that setting goals and doing them are different animals. Being realistic is key. *"In any given year, I never complete even half my goals, as I have always bitten off more than I can chew."*

Goal Setting

Use the space below to first jot down your goals. Keep in mind that they should be manageable, realistic, and achievable. Make sure that you feel "likely" or "very likely" to accomplish each goal or consider revising it.

GOAL 1 _____

Am I likely to be able to achieve this goal? (*circle one*)

  Unlikely   Somewhat Unlikely   Somewhat Likely   Likely   Very Likely

Action Plan to Accomplish Goal

_____

_____

GOAL 2 _____

Am I likely to be able to achieve this goal? (*circle one*)

  Unlikely   Somewhat Unlikely   Somewhat Likely   Likely   Very Likely

Action Plan to Accomplish Goal

_____

_____

GOAL 3 _____

Am I likely to be able to achieve this goal? (*circle one*)

  Unlikely   Somewhat Unlikely   Somewhat Likely   Likely   Very Likely

Action Plan to Accomplish Goal

_____

_____

GOAL 4 _____

Am I likely to be able to achieve this goal? (*circle one*)

  Unlikely   Somewhat Unlikely   Somewhat Likely   Likely   Very Likely

Action Plan to Accomplish Goal

_____

_____

Here's an example for you. Is one of your goals to exercise more often? Let's say you already exercise twice a week before work. You may not have given it much thought, but you have a "system" in place to enable you to do that. It may mean you wake up a little earlier on those days, lay out clothing for the morning before going to bed, and prepare lunch and snacks for you or your family the night before so that you have time to exercise. Therefore, it may be easier to tweak your existing system to add in a third day of exercise before work than trying to find a different time of day to do so. Adding goals to address your diabetes diagnosis is stressful enough. So you should try whenever possible to use your "non-diabetes" systems to help achieve those goals rather than creating new systems from scratch.

Sometimes, however, it is impossible to achieve a goal with an existing strategy and a new one needs to be created. For example, maybe you never exercised regularly before your diagnosis and now have to figure out something that will work for you. Remember: Keep it simple. We want to help you create new systems that are easy to set up but, more importantly, simple to maintain. If it is too complicated, you likely won't stick to it.

With these things in mind, now go back to your goal sheet and fill in action items that you feel will help you accomplish each goal.

Getting the Job Done

In addition to setting up systems to achieve goals, you need tactics to ensure you actually use the systems you create and reminders to keep you motivated to stay on target and continue working toward your goals. Here are some of our favorite motivational tips:

> **Write.** Write your goals down to make it more "real." Whether you write in this book or keep a list in a special notebook, journaling will help you feel accountable.

> **Post.** Posting your goals in a conspicuous place can help, especially if you are a visual person. A vision board, bulletin

Goal writing has really helped Jim Turner stay focused. *"I love to make lists of my goals. I make them for the day, week, and year. Now, as helpful as these lists are, they can sometimes start to swallow me up. When I see that happening—when I feel like I'm just accumulating goals with no intention of ever completing or even trying to complete them, I will make myself do the first thing on the list. I just do it. This is the hard part. This is the moment to make sure I jump in and DO."*

board, and even the front of the refrigerator are some great visible spots. One physician told us that she marks a red *X* on every day of her calendar that she exercises. If she sees blank days, it reminds her that she needs to get more active.

Tell. Some people are more motivated to reach their goals when they tell others about them. It makes them feel more committed. If this applies to you, then enlist the help of a friend, neighbor, or loved one. Hiring a pro, such as a professional organizer, can help you stay on track. (Visit the website of the National Association of Professional Organizers at www.NAPO.net to find an organizer near you.) Having an "account-ability" partner with whom you check in is a great way to make sure you achieve your goals.

Schedule. Break down your goals into tasks and assign a due date. Then schedule appointments with yourself to accomplish those tasks. It is much easier to stay on track when you schedule your time.

Music. For goals involving tasks that require you to stay alert and focused, consider playing music to keep you on track. Music is a great brain boost.

Reward. Don't forget to reward yourself along the way. Rewards are a wonderful motivational tool! Try an outing with a good friend, massage, or luxurious bath.

We tell our clients all the time that we don't do "perfect." We do "enough!" Organized enough. Healthy enough. Exercise enough. Achieving perfection is just not possible. Trying is only going to set you up for failure. Take the process of getting organized one step at a time. Break it down into small, manageable parts. Take on a little bit at a time. Use this book as a guide and a resource. And remember to breathe. We are with you every step of the way. You can do it!

Notes _____

_____

_____

_____

_____

_____

_____

_____

_____

_____

_____

_____

_____

_____

_____

_____

_____

_____

Overcoming Obstacles

As you begin working toward your goals, you may bump into some roadblocks that could slow you down or take you off course. On this page, you'll try to anticipate some things that may make achieving your goals more difficult and identify some personal motivational tips to keep you on track.

GOAL 1 _____

My Challenges _____

_____

What Motivates Me? _____

_____

GOAL 2 _____

My Challenges _____

_____

What Motivates Me? _____

_____

GOAL 3 _____

My Challenges _____

_____

What Motivates Me? _____

_____

GOAL 4 _____

My Challenges _____

_____

What Motivates Me? _____

_____

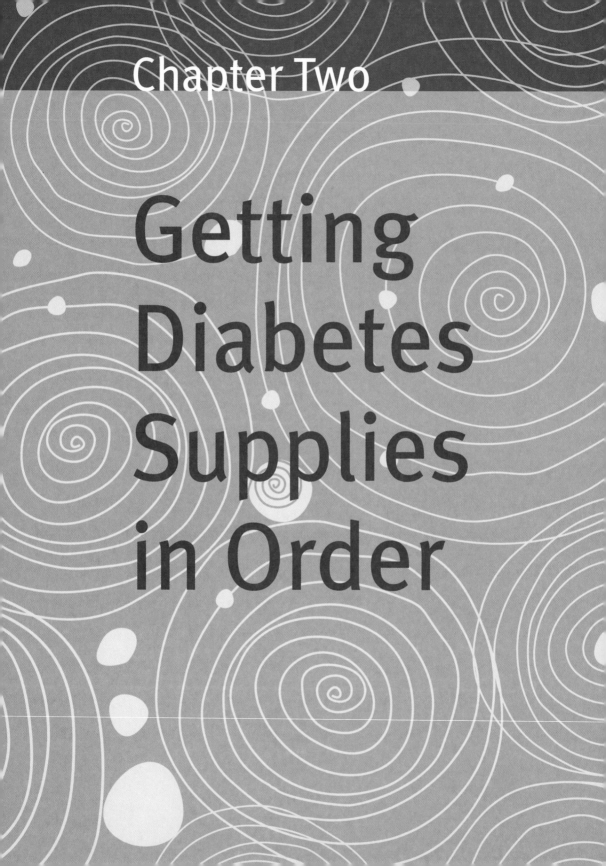

Chapter Two

Getting Diabetes Supplies in Order

A DIAGNOSIS OF DIABETES comes with a tremendous amount of supplies to manage and organize. Help! What do you do first? Don't despair. Together we can break down the process into manageable steps. Soon, you'll have an organized diabetes household. Follow us!

Diabetes Supplies Checklist

Have you ever just stared at your diabetes supplies, medications, and must-have portable snacks? Do you feel overwhelmed? Take stock of your supplies. First, create a centralized list of everything you need in order to maintain a healthy and organized diabetes life both at home and while away from home. Everyone with diabetes is different, and therefore supply needs may vary. Your medications and supplies may change over time as well.

Having one central location for a supply "brain dump" will make you feel organized immediately and take remembering what you need and have out of the equation. This list can be kept in a diabetes notebook or in a document or spreadsheet on the computer so that you don't have to worry about misplacing important supplies or information. You can access it any time or anywhere (more tips on paperwork in chapter 9).

> Remember to check expiration dates on all supplies.

Sort Your Way to Organization

Just as you sort your clothing by season or activity, you can look at your diabetes supplies in very much the same manner. Use the following sorting categories to begin to group your supplies for sensible storage.

Your daily diabetes supply list may include:

- ☐ Blood glucose meter and case
- ☐ Extra batteries
- ☐ Test strips
- ☐ Lancets and a lancet device
- ☐ Cotton balls
- ☐ Soap
- ☐ Syringe/pen, needles, or pump infusion set
- ☐ Insulin
- ☐ Oral medications
- ☐ Sharps container for safe disposal of materials
- ☐ Continuous glucose monitor (CGM) or sensor supplies
- ☐ Medical identification bracelet (or other form of ID) and identification card (kept in your wallet)
- ☐ Fast-acting source of carbohydrates (glucose tabs, gels, etc.)
- ☐ Portable snacks
- ☐ Glucagon kit
- ☐ Diabetic socks
- ☐ Food scales
- ☐ Measuring cups and spoons

Supply Categories

Supplies Needed Daily or Several Times a Day

_____

_____

Supplies Needed to Be Easily Reached

_____

_____

Supplies Requiring Refrigeration

_____

_____

Supplies to Be Kept Out of Reach of Children

_____

_____

Surplus Supplies for Storage

_____

_____

Supplies with Expiration Dates

_____

_____

Supplies to Travel with You

_____

_____

Place items that are used together in the same category. For example, your meter, test strips and lancets should be grouped together. Surplus supplies, too, can be categorized and stored together elsewhere. As you begin to look at your lists of associated supplies, you can start thinking about logical places to store each of the categories.

We asked leading diabetes blogger and creator of www.sixuntilme.com, Kerri Sparling, about how she organizes her diabetes supplies. Kerri has been living with type 1 diabetes since 1986, and she currently wears an Animas OneTouch Ping insulin pump and a Dexcom continuous glucose monitor.

According to Kerri, diabetes is a constant game of "what if?" *"Wearing an insulin pump keeps my insulin supply close at hand and constantly infusing, but I always carry emergency supplies for those just-in-case moments. I have an extra infusion set in my bag in case mine rips out. I also keep a battery on hand in case the battery needs to be replaced on my pump. And in the event of a full pump failure, I always have an insulin pen stashed in my purse. People with diabetes aren't known for traveling light.*

Since we, as people with diabetes, are always planning for the worst but hoping for the best, we do a lot of thinking ahead. Even if I'm only leaving the house for a few hours, I carry enough supplies on hand for a weekend away. It's challenging because it makes my purse the size of an airline carry-on, but the effect that insulin pumping has had on my diabetes control is worth it."

Any organizing tips for people with diabetes (PWD) who wear a pump?

"I stash my diabetes supplies like I'm channeling some insulin-deficient squirrel. In addition to keeping my standard purse armed with all the necessary accoutrements, I keep pump batteries in my wallet, extra infusion sets in my glove compartment, and my insulin pen is as handy as a regular ink pen. It seems like over-planning until you're at the movie theater and your pump is beeping for a new battery."

What do you pack your diabetes supplies in when you dash out of the house in the morning?

"My purse is not just a purse; it's a diabetes bag, a diaper bag, and oftentimes a camera bag. As a type 1 diabetic and the mother of a two-year-old, lifting my purse will give you forearms like Popeye. Thankfully, with a bag the size of Iceland, I can just throw my supplies in without worrying about taking up too much room. I could probably hide a Rottweiler in that bag."

As Kerri points out, planning and organizing are a part of everyday life with diabetes. Let's explore more specific ways to stay organized in order to manage daily blood sugars properly and help to avoid poor outcomes.

Assigning Locations

Once you have categorized your supplies, you have to decide where to put your supplies. Ask yourself the following questions. Think about them one category at a time and remember to go at your own pace. Some questions to ask yourself:

- Where do I have space in my home for my critical supplies?
- Can I relocate other items in my home to another location if necessary?
- What space do I access most so I will remember to use my supplies?
- Do I prefer to store items in drawers? Cabinets? Shelves?
- Is the space I want to use easily accessible? Well lit? Is there room for a step stool if necessary? Is it out of reach of small children?
- Can I hang hooks or a peg board to maximize the storage I need?
- Do I use essential supplies in several areas of my home? If that's the case, is "portable" storage my best option?

> Measure your designated space (depth, width, and length) before placing items in the space or before you purchase storage containers. Bring your measurements *and* tape measure with you to the store so that you purchase containers that will accommodate your supplies.

It's critical that you ask yourself these questions so that you can find an organizing solution that works for you. Don't worry if you want to store day-to-day supplies in the coat closet between the hats and scarves. We have all heard about women who use their kitchen oven to store sweaters! The only thing that matters is that the system you create works for you, is organized, and is easily maintained.

Creating Command Central

Whether it's a basement shelf or laundry-room cabinet, designate one area in your home that will function as your "command central." This is where you will store the bulk of your diabetes supplies. Remember, wherever you choose, make sure you have ample space to accommodate all the supplies.

It's All in the Containers

Whether you use open shelving or closed cabinets, shelves are the most common storage place for diabetes supplies. Open and accessible shelves are a natural and easy choice. Here are a few tips and tools for maximizing their efficiency.

- Keep supplies in clear plastic containers on a shelf. This way the container can easily be removed, necessary supplies accessed, and the container quickly put back—no miscellaneous items lost or forgotten.

> Don't have a Container Store, Walmart, or Target near you? There is no need to break the bank. Dollar stores can be your treasure trove for plastic containers in a variety of sizes and styles.

- Divide your supplies by categories to be stored in individual containers. For example
  - Keep all meter supplies together including test strips, lancets, extra batteries, and control solutions.
  - Measuring spoons, liquid and dry measuring cups, and a food scale can be stored in the kitchen. (See chapter 3 for more tips on kitchen organization.)
- For those of you who struggle with chronic disorganization and need critical items to stand out, place Velcro strips on the inside of the cabinet door and Velcro any of your essential items, such as extra batteries or alcohol wipes (if you use them), to the door. You will have all your necessities right at your fingertips.
- If you have deep shelves, think "vertical space." Drawer organizers that stack one on top of each other on a shelf are the perfect way to maximize your storage. Drawers pull out so there's no need to unstack containers to get to the ones on the bottom.
- Make sure to label each container clearly. This will act as a visual check list of what's inside.

> Make sure to keep copies of all user manuals and warranties with their corresponding equipment or in one central location. A 3-ring binder with plastic insert sheets can make a handy way to keep them all together. Better to have them handy than to have to search for them.

- If you store items on a high shelf and they are not easily reachable, keep a small folding step stool on hand for easy access.

Rolling in the Deep Drawers

Now that you have your supplies and containers in order, it's time to discuss "how-to" properly use drawer space. Deep drawers are wonderful for housing supplies as they slide out. You can see everything you have at a quick glance.

We love NACKit!, a reusable, refillable label organizing system. It uses stick-on clear vinyl pockets that stay in place, but you can change out the insert cards as many times as you need to record the container's contents. www.nackit.com

Here are our best tips to maximize your drawer space:
- Drawer dividers are the perfect solution for you to create specific sections for each category. For example, your healthy snacks, testing supplies, batteries, and wipes can all be separated by dividers.
- Designate one drawer in your kitchen for your healthy snack options. Prepackaged, single-serving snacks are best, as they are portion controlled and easily totable. You can also "baggie" your own portioned snack from a large container. You can eliminate the large packaging to create more space for a greater assortment of healthy snacks. As an added bonus, you'll be able to easily view the carbohydrate content of each snack. No guesswork necessary. Always a win-win!

- If you have deep drawers, think "air space." Baskets with high sides are the perfect way to maximize your storage.

We asked Dr. Jason Baker, an assistant professor of medicine and attending endocrinologist at Cornell Medical College in New York who has type 1 diabetes, what he recommends for storing surplus diabetes supplies. *"Rationing diabetes supplies will never result in good blood sugar control. This means keeping extra diabetes supplies (including insulin) and blood glucose meters both at home and work. If you run out of the house and forget the supplies, or your meter malfunctions, you'll still be able to properly test your blood sugar at work."* He also suggests keeping an extra supply of needles and strips in the office, so you'll never run out of these necessary materials.

Dr. Baker is the founder and director of Marjorie's Fund, www.marjoriesfund.org. The mission of Marjorie's Fund: The Type 1 Diabetes Global Initiative is to empower people living with type 1 diabetes in resource-poor settings to survive diagnosis and thrive into adulthood.

Keeping It Cold

Nonperishable, diabetes-friendly snacks can be kept in a designated drawer, but what about diabetes supplies that need to be maintained at a certain temperature? Most of your diabetes supplies should keep well as long as they are stored in a cool, dark place and are protected from direct sunlight and high temperatures. However, it is critical that insulin, food supplies, and similar items are stored at the proper temperature. Some items are best stored in the refrigerator.

Follow these tips for the optimal refrigerated storage:

- Keep diabetes-related supplies that need to be kept cool in separate, plastic food storage containers. Pick storage containers that you designate solely for your diabetes supplies and make sure that everything is properly labeled. This will ensure that your supplies don't migrate to the back of the fridge behind the milk or condiments.
- Keep all refrigerated medical supplies in the same place. Use a compartment that is easily accessible, such as any empty fruit or vegetable drawer or the butter compartment. You can store your insulin in the butter compartment as that area gives you

IKEA's line of Rationell drawer dividers accommodates extra deep drawers that are up to 36" wide. For more standard dividers, try the Container Store, Bed Bath & Beyond, or Target.

Healthy snacks are essential supplies for people with diabetes so we asked Toby Smithson, a registered dietitian-nutritionist and certified diabetes educator, for some snacking tips. Toby is a spokesperson for the Academy of Nutrition and Dietetics and the creator of everydaydiabetes.com, a website devoted to living well with diabetes. She has successfully managed her own diabetes for the past 43 years.

According to Toby, *"Organized snacking is essential for good blood sugar management. If you don't have the right foods with you, chances are you will be tempted to grab a less healthy option."*

Toby's top picks for portable snacks are *"fiber-rich bars because they are easy to carry, prewrapped, preportioned, and contain a food label as a reminder of how many carbohydrates are in the bar. They also contain fiber to slow down carbohydrate absorption, which helps reduce spikes in blood sugar levels. These snacks should be stashed around the house, office, and car, and in your bag so they are easily accessible."* She reminds us not to rely solely on fiber bars for our total daily fiber intake. Toby adds, *"I carry the lower carbohydrate mini snack bars that* use slowly digestible carbohydrates, which help to reduce blood sugar spikes."

When we asked Toby for recommendations to curb hunger when in normal blood sugar range, she suggested shelled peanuts or almonds. *"Nuts contain healthy fats and are low in carbohydrates, which helps to control blood sugar. Reducing simple carbohydrates, spreading carbohydrates throughout the day, and eating protein and healthy fats (such as unsalted nuts) will help keep your weight in check and improve blood sugar control."* She recommends carrying portioned nuts in a resealable plastic bag or tin.

the cold of the refrigerator and is easily accessible.

- Make sure all of your diabetes supplies are kept up to date. Regularly check all expiration dates. Just as you would maintain an inventory of food in your pantry, rotating the older food to the front and placing the newer food to the back to eliminate waste, the same should be done for medications and any supplies that have expiration dates.

> A brightly colored lid makes diabetes supplies easy to spot. Tupperware and Rubbermaid make containers with fun, colorful lids that fit tightly.

- For snacks that might need to be refrigerated (or that you prefer to refrigerate), such as juice boxes, puddings, or other to-go snacks, use the same system as you would for either a shelf or drawer. Empty the items from their original wrapping or packaging to create a quick "grab and go" section.
- Label, Label, Label. Anything you store in the refrigerator needs to be properly labeled so you are clear on expiration dates.
- Does it seem as if you don't have room for containers in your refrigerator? Large clear plastic storage bags work quite well. Make sure to purchase ones that have a strong closing mechanism. We like the bags with the sliding zipper enclosures best. They prevent air from getting in and contents from spilling out. Again, keep them all in one spot in the refrigerator.

Dr. Jason Baker advises his patients, *"Always look at the expiration date on a new bottle of insulin prior to using it, and only use a vial of insulin for one month prior to changing to a new one. This helps to ensure the insulin continues to perform properly."* As Dr. Baker has type 1 diabetes himself, he is acutely aware of the importance of storing insulin. He recommends keeping insulin that is not currently in use in an area of the refrigerator where you are assured that freezing will not occur (such as a vegetable crisper drawer). *"Keep the insulin where you can eyeball it periodically to see if the supply is running too low,"* says Dr. Baker. For insulin that is currently being used, he recommends keeping both a vial of basal/bolus (or an extra vile of bolus if on a pump) in your meter case at room temperature. *"Don't carry the insulin in your pocket or leave it in the heat (in the sun or near a space heater) or in a very cold environment. Remember that insulin can denature more quickly at extreme temperatures. Also, keep diabetes supplies in stock. If you are ordering something online, it's important to make sure that you have enough of a supply at home while you await your next delivery."*

- Clearly label contents or expiration dates right on the bag. No guesswork involved.

Short on Space

Do you have limited storage space? Let's explore improved space management for your supplies. Not everyone has the space to store all their necessary kitchen, cooking, or diabetes supplies. Kitchen drawers can be tiny and pantry shelf space may be tight. Time to get creative! Here are our tried and true tips on how you can maximize small spaces.

- If you are limited on space, purchase small plastic drawers that can sit on top of a counter in the kitchen or a dresser in the bedroom. Alcohol wipes, needles, lancets, carbohydrate counting

> Keep markers and labels nearby so you can label as you store. This way you will eliminate the need to search through the house when you are putting items away.

> The Container Store and Target are our go-to spots for stacking drawers. You can find everything from single deep drawer styles to five-drawer mini-stacking series. Find the best one to fit your space and needs.

book, etc. will all fit nicely in the mini-drawer units. Extra meters, ketone strips, and the like will fill up a larger size.

- Have ample storage in the basement or laundry room? Then store your excess medical supplies in a large Rubbermaid cabinet or tote box. Make sure the lid seals tightly.

- If you are really tight on space, bring your walls into play. Hang a peg board or no-fuss shelving on an empty wall—perfect for a laundry room, bathroom, or kitchen. This is a natural storage solution for snacks or supplies. For those who suffer from "out-of-sight, out-of-mind" syndrome, this method keeps critical items at your fingertips.

- Have ample hanging space in your closets but short on shelves? Hang a clear shoe storage bag in your closet and tuck snacks, testing equipment, supplies, etc. in the pockets. Hanging sweater or shirt storage bags works just as well for bigger supplies.

> IKEA has inexpensive peg boards in their kitchen section. Remember to think "outside the box" when you want to create space. Scour office supply and craft stores for workable solutions.

Locating storage areas in your home is almost like embarking on a treasure hunt. Begin by searching through rooms in your house to identify available options. Be creative in the way you consider your environment and you should be able to come up with some great ideas. Consider what things aren't utilized as often to see what areas can be freed up. For example, could moving china used once or twice a year to a basement storage cabinet free up a valuable kitchen location for supplies used every day?

With your list of supplies in need of storage in hand, grab a tape measure and explore. After you've identified and measured your available supply locations, visit kitchen and office supply stores to locate some amazing containers to fit your needs and spaces. By following our recommendations for creative and effective storage solutions, you will have your home organized in no time!

Notes _____

_____

_____

_____

_____

_____

_____

_____

_____

_____

_____

_____

Consider Your Storage Options

Storage location 1 _____
Possible storage for: _____
Dimensions: _____ (length) _____ (width) _____ (height)
Limitations: _____

Storage location 2 _____
Possible storage for: _____
Dimensions: _____ (length) _____ (width) _____ (height)
Limitations: _____

Storage location 3 _____
Possible storage for: _____
Dimensions: _____ (length) _____ (width) _____ (height)
Limitations: _____

Storage location 4 _____
Possible storage for: _____
Dimensions: _____ (length) _____ (width) _____ (height)
Limitations: _____

Storage location 5 _____
Possible storage for: _____
Dimensions: _____ (length) _____ (width) _____ (height)
Limitations: _____

Chapter Three

Your Diabetes-Friendly Kitchen

HAS A MEMBER OF YOUR HEALTHCARE TEAM ever asked you to eat nutritious and well-balanced meals? Has your doctor or registered dietitian-nutritionist "strongly suggested" that you eat less sugary, processed, and fast foods? You probably already know that you can improve your blood sugar levels and possibly prevent diabetes complications if you eat well and take care of yourself. You may have thought about preparing and consuming more lean proteins (such as fish, chicken, and turkey) and whole grains, along with plenty of vegetables. Your doctor might have suggested different ways to help control your blood sugar level with diet. Perhaps you're familiar with carb counting or have used the glycemic index to help control your blood sugar levels. If you were diagnosed with diabetes a few years ago, you might have even followed a diabetes food exchange list. Maybe you've even read a book or two on how to eat well and control your blood sugar when you have diabetes.

For more information on carb counting, visit www.diabetes.org/food-and-fitness/food/planning-meals/carb-counting/ Glycemic index information can be found at www.diabetes.org/food-and-fitness/food/planning-meals/glycemic-index-and-diabetes.html

In your research, have you noticed that many food and nutrition experts recommend that you prepare most of your meals at home?

In fact, medical experts suggest that you eat healthy well-balanced meals whether or not you have diabetes. If you or a loved one has been diagnosed with diabetes, frequent meal preparation will likely become part of your family's healthy lifestyle.

Take a moment and think about why you might not want to cook at home. Is it because your kitchen is disorganized? No matter what approach you take toward healthier eating, an organized kitchen will help to increase your confidence when it comes to meal preparation. Your kitchen typically gets more use (and abuse) than any other room in your home. Whether you want to prepare a leisurely family dinner or a grab-and-go breakfast, you can do both more easily with a more organized kitchen. If you properly arrange your food, pots, pans, utensils, and measuring tools, you'll be able to cook with ease. In this chapter, we will guide you through the basic steps you need to organize your kitchen. Don't feel overwhelmed in your kitchen, we're here to help!

Set Up Your Kitchen's Organizing System

Think about your kitchen's condition *before* you were diagnosed with diabetes. Was your kitchen camera-ready for a photo spread in *Architectural Digest* or filled with clutter? Are you now faced with the challenge of how to conveniently store your diabetes testing supplies as well as traditional food items? What about meal preparation tools? By following our strategies and guidelines, you can set up a workable kitchen that is both organized and easy to maintain. You'll be able to find everything you need to properly manage your diabetes and prepare healthy meals in record time!

Robin Plotkin, RD, LD, a culinary nutritionist and health blogger, says, *"If organizing the kitchen isn't your niche, ask someone you think has an amazingly organized kitchen to come in with a critical eye to help you with this step. It can be overwhelming, but with a little support, it's much more manageable."* Great advice, Robin!

A Fresh Eye

The first step to set up your kitchen properly is to take a look at each existing organizational system with a fresh eye. We know that the most difficult part for you is to get started. Don't worry! Ask yourself one question at a time. Feel free to move at your own pace, and, please, take your time. After you feel satisfied with your response to one question, move on to the next.

Ask yourself the following questions:

Where is the best place to store my essential diabetes supplies?

_____

Can I find the ingredients and cookware that I need to prepare healthy and delicious meals?

_____

Does kitchen clutter litter my countertops? Does the clutter make healthy food preparation a challenge?

_____

Is my kitchen organized by "fit," rather than "use"? For example, is your mixed nut jar in a back corner of your kitchen counter because it fits there, even though you and your family reach for it multiple times each day?

_____

Are my pots and pans easily accessible? Or, do I have to reach and sort through them every time I need to use one?

_____

Are my pantry items grouped by "like with like"? Spices in one zone? Cereals in another?

_____

Am I using the items in my kitchen on a regular basis? Or can I relocate some items elsewhere?

_____

Are the items in my pantry and on my cabinet shelves easily accessible? Is everything that I need to prepare well-balanced meals visible? Do I actually know what is in my pantry and cabinets?

_____

After you answer each of these questions, you can begin to figure out what areas of your kitchen are "organizationally challenged." Take a step-by-step approach to help you decide whether or not you need to make major adjustments or small tweaks to your current kitchen organization system. Let's put our heads together and figure out what solutions work best for you.

Now that you've spent some time considering the challenges in your kitchen, you can start to take some steps to maximize your kitchen space. Select one idea below at a time. Come back to this page when you are ready to try another tip. Don't worry if an idea or tool doesn't work for you at this moment; you can always come back to this detailed list whenever you are ready.

Organizing Storage Spaces

No matter what state your kitchen might be in, chances are you can benefit from adopting a few organizing strategies. We know that some kitchens are very small and space is limited, but even in larger kitchens space always seems to be at a premium. For that reason, it makes sense to go through the items in the kitchen to be sure they all still belong there. Consider the following key organizing concepts:

Toss anything that is broken, chipped, expired, rusty, or missing parts. These items are huge "space robbers" and take up valuable real estate.

Donate never-used small appliances and gadgets, gently used gifts, extra plastic ware, jars, and items you no longer like, want, or need. Instant space!

Move seldom-used items such as holiday dishes or party platters to either a high, out-of-the-way shelf or other location in your home, such as a basement or garage.

Group related items together. For example, keep all quick-acting carbohydrate sources together in a drawer or on an easy-to-reach shelf. Make sure you can get to these items easily in case you have a low blood sugar. This will also help you cut down on duplicate purchases.

Create Space in already existing shelves, cabinets, and pantry closets.

Tips and Tools for Creating Space

Here are some of our favorite organizing tools for creating space in the kitchen.

> Check out IKEA's Variera shelves to add to an existing shelf to double storage space.

- Place wire shelf expanders on cabinet shelves to double storage capacity.
- Use graduated risers (like mini-steps or stairs) in pantries to hold spices and canned goods.
- Go behind closed doors! Hang door-mounted racks on the inside of pantry closets or cabinet doors to maximize storage space. This is a great technique for freeing up counter space.

> For an inexpensive and flexible option, you can hang a clear plastic shoe bag to the inside of your pantry door. Perfect for corralling your meter and testing supplies or baggies with preportioned snacks (check out the list later in the chapter for suggestions).

- Install sliding baskets under the sink or on a deep shelf to store those hard-to-reach items. This makes those back-of-cabinet items instantly accessible.
- Think "air space" and mount a ceiling rack for pots and pans. Imagine how much easier (and quieter) it will be to reach for a pan you need when it's hanging from its own hook. Now you won't have to rummage and rattle through a pile of pans to get to the one you need.
- Turn it around! Installing Lazy Susans and plastic turntables in deep or corner cabinets lets you have everything right at your fingertips.
- Keep the items you use most regularly in your prime pantry real estate. This means the space between your shoulders and knees. Now that makes sense!
- Lid baskets or drying racks are simple solutions for keeping all your pot lids together. Allows you to grab the right size lid in seconds.
- Peg boards are a fun and efficient way to maximize space. Hang one by the stove to hold cooking utensils, oven mitts, knives, and other everyday items.
- Short on space? Purchase a rolling cart with ample storage space to house items you use frequently. Then store the cart out of the

> No need to break the bank when hunting down kitchen organizing supplies. Dollar and odd-lot type stores are a treasure trove for containers, bins, and baskets.

way when not in use. Look for ones with a butcher block top to give you an additional cutting and chopping zone.

- Use expandable drawer dividers in your silverware, utensil, and junk drawer. Every home is allowed one!

By improving the organization of your kitchen, you can both cut the time it takes to prepare your healthy meals and snacks and make that time spent there more enjoyable and less stressful. Once you get started, we bet you'll even find your own favorite tips and products.

Whitmor's Expanding Drawer Dividers come in sets of two and can be used front-to-back or side-to-side. They also expand to 21.75"! (www.holdnstorage.com)

Apps for the Kitchen

Topic	iPhone	Android
Carb Count	Carb Counting with Lenny, Eat Smart with Hope Warshaw, Diabetes Nutrition by Fooducate	Carb Counting with Lenny, Eat Smart with Hope Warshaw, Fooducate
Cooking	Salad Secrets, iCookbook Diabetic, Big Oven, Evernote Food, iPhoto Cookbook, Mark Bittman How to Cook Everything Essentials, Drag 'n Cook	Big Oven, Evernote Food, Diabetic Audio Recipes Chef Tap, MyCookbook: Cooking Basics Recipe Search
Pantry	Notes, BugMe!, Notability, Best Before	Notes, BugMe!, Colornote, My Pantry, Best Before
Refrigerator	Consume Within, Leftovers, Best Before	Best Before, Food Expiration Saver, Stinky Food
Food Safety	Food Safety at Home, USDA Food Safety (not by USDA), Is My Food Safe? (AND)	Is My Food Safe? (AND)
Grocery Shop	Grocery Guru, Grocery IQ, Out of Milk, Diabetes Fooducate, Smarter Shopping, iAteGreat, Seafood Watch, Smarter Shopping with Phil Lempert	Grocery Guru, Grocery IQ, Out of Milk, ToMarket Grocery Shopping, Grocery Smart-Shopping List
Spices	iSpice, Culinary Herbs & Spice Encyclopedia	iSpice, Culinary Herbs & Spice Bible
Produce	Markon's Produce Guide, Fresh Fruit, Food Focus: Fruits game, Veggie Garden Palooza game	Markon's Produce Guide
Diabetes Drawer	Glucagon	Glucool Diabetes Premium
Organizations	Diabetes Forecast (ADA), Pocket First Aid & CPR (AHA)	Diabetes Forecast (ADA), Pocket First Aid & CPR (AHA)

Source: Adapted from *An App A Day* and *An App A Day for Health Professionals*, © 2012, Frederico Arts LLC; www.AppyLiving.com.

Here are our suggestions for some prepackaged nutritious snacks that contain less than 20 grams of carbohydrates. Do not eat too many packaged snacks as they may contain a lot of sodium. Moderation is key!

Snack Description	Manufacturer	Serving Size	Energy (kcal)	CHO (g)	Protein (g)	Fiber (g)
Peach Chunks Fruit Naturals, No Sugar Added	Del Monte	½ cup	40	12	1	2
Breast of Chicken in Water, No Salt Added	Hormel	56 g	45	0	9	0
Chunk Light Tuna in Water, 50% Less Sodium	Chicken of the Sea	2 oz	50	0	11	0
Solid White Albacore Tuna in Water	StarKist	3 oz	110	<1	21	<1
Sugar Free Pudding	Jell-O	160 g snack pack	60	13	1	1
Pineapple Tidbits in Pineapple Juice	Dole	122 g	60	15	1	<1
Chocolate Crunch Rice Cakes	Quaker	1 cake	60	12	1	0
Healthy Picks Blueberry Pomegranate Applesauce, No Sugar Added	Musselman's	4 oz	70	17	0	3
Dried Wasabi Peas	Trader Joe's	⅓ cup	80	12	1	1
Harvest Cheddar 100 Calorie Mini Bites	Sun Chips	1 bag	100	12	2	1
Emerald Natural Walnuts and Almonds 100 Calorie Pack	Diamond of California	1 pack	100	3	3	1

Snack Description	Manufacturer	Serving Size	Energy (kcal)	CHO (g)	Protein (g)	Fiber (g)
Cheddar Goldfish Baked Snack Crackers 100 Calorie Pack	Pepperidge Farm	1 pack	100	14	3	1
Living Fiber Fit Oatmeal Chocolate Chunk Cookies	Kraft— South Beach	1 pack	100	17	5	1
Cinnamon Roll Thin Crisps	Honey Maid	1 bag	100	16	1	0
Gourmet Lite White Half Salt Popcorn	Vic's	3 cups	110	18	3	4
Rich Cheddar Cheese Soy Crisps	Genisoy	17 crisps	120	13	7	2
Baked Cheddar Snack Mix	Quaker	¾ cup	130	19	2	1
All Natural Old Style Picture Show Microwave Popcorn	Newman's Own	3½ cups	130	18	2	3
Cinnamon Crisps	Extend	1 bag (32 g)	130	17	8	3
Blue Corn Tortilla Chips	Garden of Eatin'	28 g (about 16 chips)	140	18	2	2
Natural Yellow Corn Chips	Tostitos	28 g	150	19	2	1
Harvest Dark Chocolate Forest Blend	Planters	¼ cup	170	18	4	3
Trail Mix, Feel 'N Healthy Mix	Good Sense	¼ cup	180	13	6	3
Uber Roasted Nut Roll	Lara Bar	14	220	14	5	2

Kitchen Challenge

What are your favorite kitchen organizational tips?

_____

_____

_____

_____

_____

_____

_____

_____

_____

_____

_____

_____

_____

Notes

Chapter Four

The Organized Refrigerator, Freezer, and Pantry

YES, IT'S TIME to take a peek inside your refrigerator and freezer. You will need that space to store healthy food along with diabetes medications and supplies that require refrigeration (such as insulin in the refrigerator and ice packs in the freezer). Don't wait until you start your spring cleaning to give your refrigerator and freezer a thorough clean out. Now is the time to organize your kitchen storage space! With our easy step-by-step instructions, you will have a clean, orderly, and useable refrigerator.

The Big Clean

A well-organized refrigerator is necessary if your goal is to prepare nutritious meals and improve your blood sugar control. However, all of our tips and tools apply to anyone who wants to have a "healthy" refrigerator. Remember, start with one step at a time, but read through our tips several times before you get started. This process will take some time, so please don't rush. We are right here with you!

Let's start at the very beginning.
1. Gather up several heavy garbage bags and a recycling container for the glassware, jars, and cans. If you haven't cleaned the inside of your refrigerator and freezer in a while, have your cleaning supplies at the ready.
2. Empty out the entire contents of the refrigerator and freezer. Keep a clean cooler with ice packs on the kitchen table to store cold foods while you clean. Toss anything that is expired,

freezer-burned, spoiled, or moldy. If the container hosting the food is questionable, toss it along with the spoiled food. You know the old saying "when in doubt, throw it out."

3. Move the refrigerator away from the wall and wipe away any dust, dirt, or old food particles from the wall behind and floor beneath.

4. Scrub the inside of the refrigerator and freezer with warm, soapy water. Don't just wash the areas that have puddles and spills; the pull-out baskets and drawers need to be washed, too! Dry the inside of the refrigerator thoroughly with paper towels or clean cloths.

5. Place a "refrigerator-friendly" baking soda freshener in the back of the refrigerator to capture lingering odors.

6. Test the refrigerator thermometer. The temperature should be set for less than 40 degrees in the refrigerator and 0 degrees in the freezer. If for any reason your temperatures are registering too high or too low, consult your user's manual or contact a service repairman right away.

You've done it! You now have a clean refrigerator. You are ready to start restocking. Good for you!

For more kitchen safety tips from Food Safety and Inspection Service, visit www.fsis.usda.gov/PDF/Kitchen_Companion.pdf

Refrigerator Restock

Now that you have a clean, temperature-controlled refrigerator and freezer, it's time to put your food away. Where does everything go? Make sure to arrange the refrigerator to your likes and needs. YOU need to be comfortable with how your refrigerator is arranged. Now that you have an organized and useable refrigerator, you can start to prepare healthy and well-balanced meals. After all, if you can't find a food or ingredient for a diabetes-friendly recipe, you can't prepare it!

Make sure to read over our suggestions a few times before you begin the restocking process. It may seem a bit detailed at first glance. Don't worry! Go at your own pace. Soon you'll have an organized and well-stocked refrigerator.

Ready? Set? Restock!

- Check to see if your refrigerator shelves are adjustable. Move shelves around to make room for your large bottles of seltzers, milk, or bottled waters.
- When you place items back in the refrigerator, make sure to leave room for air to circulate. Proper air flow helps to keep food at its freshest.
- Group like items together. Yogurts and cheeses. Condiments and sauces. You get the idea! This will make your ability to find ingredients a breeze and cut down on duplicate purchases.
- Create a basket of refrigerated diabetes-friendly snacks.

- Keep Greek yogurt and hummus in a clear container so you have healthy food choices right at your fingertips.
- Put condiments, such as salad dressing and soy sauce, on the inside of the refrigerator door or on a Lazy Susan. Keep only one of each item in the refrigerator to maximize space.
- Store butter in your refrigerator's designated shelf (if there is one). This helps keep butter at its optimum temperature. Or, you might store your insulin in this compartment instead. Your choice.

We love the refrigerator cubes by Fridge Binz. See-through and multi-sized, they are perfect for your refrigerator or pantry items. Look for them online.

Robin Plotkin, RD, LD, culinary nutritionist and health blogger says, *"When diagnosed with gestational diabetes, I found it helpful to turn all condiment bottles around so that I could quickly glance at the carbohydrate content. They stayed this way for only a few weeks. By then, I had memorized them! I also took a permanent marker to all food and drink containers/cartons, etc. and wrote the grams of carbohydrates in large numbers on the front. That way, I could quickly see what had the right number of carbs I needed for that particular meal or snack."*

- Did you know that a refrigerator's temperature is at its highest on the top shelf? Keep items that don't need to be very cold on that shelf, such as calorie-free soda, bottled waters, and seltzer.
- Keep cold cuts and hard cheeses in a designated drawer. If you do not have a drawer in your refrigerator, place them in clear glass or plastic containers on a lower shelf.
- If you have the space, store your fruits and vegetables in separate refrigerator drawers. Some fruits and vegetables give off ethylene gas, which speeds up the ripening process. If you store your veggies and fruits together, some may spoil before their time.
- Make sure to store all produce in perforated bags. You can simply punch holes (about an inch apart) in plastic bags for this purpose. Don't wash your vegetables until you're ready to use them, as this will extend their shelf life.
- Wrap raw meats in plastic or aluminum foil to keep these items at their optimum freshness. Keep raw meats, poultry, and seafood on the bottom shelf of the refrigerator. Never place raw meat

Keep tomatoes, onions, sweet potatoes, bananas, avocados, and garlic in the pantry or on the counter out of direct sunlight. This will help them stay fresh and maintain their delicious taste. Other fruits, such as melon and pineapple, should only be refrigerated after they are cut.

above cooked food. Proper storage placement can help prevent meat drippings from contaminating already cooked foods. Food safety is very important!

> **Purchase freezer bags with zippered closures to keep food fresh longer!**

- Use plastic freezer bags to protect foods from freezer burn. Most bags have a place on them to clearly mark contents and dates. If you plan to purchase ahead and freeze regularly, you may want to buy one of the vacuum storage units.

- See-through storage containers are perfect for storing leftovers in either the fridge or freezer. These containers can help you easily identify leftovers. You can see the contents without lifting the lids. Extra bonus? Use containers that go easily from fridge to freezer and from microwave to dishwasher.

- Freeze foods in individual portions. You can defrost what you want and eat whenever you are ready.

- Remember to properly refrigerate your insulin vials and pens (see chapter 2). NEVER keep these supplies in the back of the refrigerator where they can't be seen!

- Most people don't have time to cook every night. So, when you do cook, try to cook enough for at least one extra dinner. Properly using leftovers is a great way to stay on your healthy eating plan. We discuss this concept in more detail in chapter 7.

Calling the kitchen his second home, Chef Sam Talbot, of *The Sweet Life: Diabetes Without Boundaries*, "dishes" on his never fail tips for maintaining a diabetes-friendly kitchen. One of his favorites is grouping like items together. "*I keep my alternative flours together—coconut flour, chickpea flour, flax meal, almond meal, etc. Nuts, legumes, and seeds go together; oils, vinegars, mustards, and cooking bases stay together as well as my cereals and grains.*" Chef Talbot also recommends that you keep a low blood sugar section in a drawer in the fridge with natural juices and candies that crunch easily. "*I don't keep refined foods in my cabinets at all, except maybe some type of granola bars for quick and easy energy. I also use the first-in first-out system (FIFO), so my fresh produce, juices, and meats are always easy to find and use quickly.*"

Keep less healthy snacks (such as salty chips or cookies) on a higher pantry shelf. That way, you will be less tempted to snack on junk food.

The healthiest foods in your refrigerator don't improve your diet if they spoil before you use them. And, particularly vegetables and fruits lose a good share of their nutritional value if they sit around too long. Take a minute to think back through items from your refrigerator you have thrown away in the last month. What would be a better quantity to purchase on future trips to the store? Both your diet and your pocketbook will thank you on this one!

Discarded Item	Purchase Quantity

Organize Leftovers

Leftovers can quickly get out of hand and become hard to identify over time. Designate one shelf or container in your refrigerator just for leftovers. That way you'll be able to prevent them from getting lost in a "black hole" in the back of the refrigerator. Label, label, label. Use masking tape and markers or erasable food storage labels to record the contents and date that each food was prepared. Make sure you label a dish before you put it away. This way you'll know when to dispose of a particular food item. Soon you'll be able to minimize un-

Robin Plotkin says, *"I leave a marker and tape on top of the fridge. That way, I just have to reach up when I' m ready to label my leftovers!"*

necessary waste and keep your refrigerator organized. Check out guidelines for tossing leftovers at www.foodsafety.gov/keep/charts/storagetimes.html.

Your Diabetes-Friendly Refrigerator and Freezer

Check in your newly clean refrigerator and freezer to see how many of these healthy foods you find there and then pick up some additional ones on your next trip to the grocery store.

- [ ] Fresh lean protein—fish, chicken, turkey (whole or ground), lean beef or pork
- [ ] Chia and hemp seeds
- [ ] Eggs
- [ ] Fresh fish
- [ ] Fresh seasonal fruit—apples, berries, cherries, freshly cut cantaloupe, grapefruit, grapes, honeydew melon, kiwi, oranges, peaches, pears, pineapples, plums, tangerines, and watermelon (to name just a few—pick your favorites!)
- [ ] Fresh vegetables—asparagus, broccoli, cabbage, carrots, cauliflower, cucumber, edamame (soy beans), eggplant, green beans, lettuces, peppers, radishes, snow peas, spinach, squashes, sugar snap peas (same as fruits, no bad choices here!)
- [ ] Frozen fruits and vegetables
- [ ] Frozen lean proteins—egg substitutes, salmon, tilapia, tuna

Your Diabetes-Friendly Refrigerator and Freezer

- [ ] Ground flaxseed to sprinkle over breakfast cereal, fruit, sandwiches, smoothies, and yogurt for extra omega-3 fatty acids
- [ ] Horseradish
- [ ] Hot sauce
- [ ] Hummus
- [ ] Low-fat dairy—skim or 1% fat string cheese (part-skim mozzarella), Greek yogurt, low-fat cottage cheese, low-fat soy or almond milk, skim or 1% milk
- [ ] Low-fat salad dressings
- [ ] Meat substitutes/soy products/tofu
- [ ] Mushrooms
- [ ] Mustard, low-sodium soy sauce, mayonnaise
- [ ] Salsa
- [ ] Pickles
- [ ] Try to buy local and in-season produce. If fresh produce is not readily available, stock up on frozen or low-sodium canned.

Let's Go Food Shopping

Here are our tried and true guidelines for food shopping success.

Prepare your food shopping list with a goal of good blood sugar control in mind. Do you need to purchase lean protein foods (such as chicken or fish) and more veggies, almonds, and hummus? Or, do you have plenty already for the week ahead? It is much more convenient to shop when you have a guide to get you through the store. Take along your handwritten notes or use one of the many new food shopping apps available for your phone.

> Check your blood sugar before you food shop to make sure you are not hypoglycemic. Remember to never go to the supermarket hungry or you are likely to purchase foods you don't want or need!

Do your homework before going to the store. Food and nutrition labels are available online for most food items. Do your research beforehand. Pay close attention to serving sizes. Look for foods with recognizable ingredients listed first (such as whole grains). Avoid foods that list sugar, dextrose, or high-fructose corn syrup in the first five ingredients.

Map your route through the supermarket before you leave home. Avoid unhealthy purchases by primarily shopping the outer perimeter of the store where the fresh fruits, vegetables, meats, and dairy foods are located.

70

> Chef Talbot recommends making a shopping list with the whole family so everyone is on the same page. *"Pick a number of recipes for the week and buy only those needed items. Then do a snack list that keeps your snack ideas all together. Keep it simple and consistent and stay away from packaged, processed, 'cardboard' food."*

Clip coupons. Coupons—online and in newspapers—save you money on healthy items and staples, such as frozen vegetables and canned goods. Most stores also have free "club cards" that provide automatic discounts. Make sure to sign up for your store's program.

Avoid temptations. Supermarkets are designed so that you purchase items you don't want or need. Stay clear of the last minute purchases at the checkout. Those impulse buys will put you over your financial and carbohydrate budget. Stick to your shopping list to avoid extra purchases and pounds!

Resist "BLTs"—bites, licks, and tastes. Those unportioned samples offered at warehouse stores or specialty grocers are usually frozen foods laden with excess salt, fat, and carbohydrates that can raise your blood sugar and pack on the pounds. Be careful, those calories and carbohydrate grams will add up quickly.

Shop online! Have your groceries delivered right to your doorstep. Plan your meals and snacks for the week and purchase everything you need with a click of a button. Most stores now have weekly circulars available online, so you can check out sales on your smartphone or computer.

Pack your groceries correctly. Keep all refrigerated, frozen, and pantry items together when packing bags at the checkout line. This will make unpacking groceries convenient and quick.

Hot items need to cool off a bit before placing them in the refrigerator. Take lids off to cool hot foods quickly and use shallow containers for storage. You should get hot foods into the refrigerator within two hours to prevent bacterial growth.

Be a detective and look for sugar's "other names" in your food.

Agave nectar	Evaporated cane juice	Lactose
Barley malt		Malt
Beet sugar	Free-flowing brown sugars	Maltose
Brown sugar		Malt syrup
Buttered syrup	Fructose	Molasses
Cane crystals	Fruit juice concentrates	Powdered sugar
Cane sugar		Raw sugar
Corn sweetener	Glucose	Rice syrup
Corn syrup	High-fructose corn syrup	Sucrose
Date sugar		Syrup
Demerara sugar	Honey	Turbinado sugar
Dextrose	Invert sugar	Yellow sugar

Reading Nutrition Labels

Learning to read a nutrition label is a key step toward improving your diet.

Nutrition Facts

❶ Serving Size 1/2 cup (115g)
Servings Per Container About 4

Amount Per Serving

❷ Calories 250   Calories from Fat 130

                                % Daily Value* ❹

Total Fat 14g	**22%**
Saturated Fat 9g	45%
Cholesterol 55mg	**18%**
Sodium 75mg	**3%**
❸ **Total Carbohydrate** 26g	**9%**
Dietary Fiber 0g	0%
Sugars 26g	
Protein 4g	

Vitamin A 10%	Vitamin C 0%
Calcium 10%	Iron 0%

* Percent Daily Values are based on a 2,000 calorie diet.

1. Check out the serving size. You may be surprised to find that the serving size is very different from what you are used to eating. If a serving size is one cup, but you usually eat two cups, you will need to double all the other values on the food label, including calories. Serving sizes may be different from what you might consider normal if you follow carbohydrate exchanges.

2. Check out the calories per serving. Generally speaking, 40 calories per serving is considered low, 100 calories is moderate, and 400 calories is high. Remember to multiply the calories by the number of servings you are actually eating.

3. Pay attention to total carbohydrates, not total sugars. Both natural and added sugars are already included in the total carbohydrate amount. One carb exchange is 15 grams, so divide the total carbohydrates by 15 if you are following an exchange plan.

4. The nutrition label contains % Daily Value (%DV). The %DV is based on consuming 2,000 calories per day. You may need fewer or more calories, but the %DV still gives you a good idea of whether the food is low or high in certain nutrients. Less than 5% DV is low,

and greater than 20% DV is high. Use these percentages to help you limit total fat, saturated fat, trans fat, cholesterol, and sodium. Look for a high %DV in calcium, iron, vitamins A and C, and fiber, which will help stabilize your blood sugar. A "good source" of a nutrient will have at least 10% DV and a high fiber food has at least 5 grams of fiber/serving.

Lastly, consider the ingredients, which are listed by weight, from the largest to the smallest amount. Try to avoid foods with sugar, dextrose, or high-fructose corn syrup in the first five ingredients. Remember that a label can say zero trans fat but the food may still have less than 0.5 grams trans fat per serving, so check the ingredients for partially hydrogenated oils. Look for ingredients you can actually pronounce!

Meal Preparation

How many times have you started to prepare a high-protein, high-fiber, carbohydrate-conscious meal only to find you are missing an ingredient? Or, have you been in a situation where you can't find the pot you need? Or you still need to wash and chop your fresh broccoli, red peppers, and scallions for your delicious chicken recipe, but you forgot to defrost the chicken? We've all been there.

Have you ever heard of the term *mise en place? Mise en place* (MEEZ ahn plahs) is a French term that means "put in place" or "everything has a place." Professional chefs as well as home cooks use the concept of *mise en place* to gather, prepare, and organize their ingredients *before*

Websites and Apps to Make Shopping a Breeze

Carb Counting Carb Counting with Lenny, Eat Smart with Hope Warshaw, Diabetes Nutrition by Fooducate, MyNetDiary, Carbs and Cals

Cooking Salad Secrets, iCookbook Diabetic, Big Oven, iPhoto Cookbook, Mark Bittman's How to Cook Everything Essentials, Drag 'n Cook, Evernote Food, Figwee, Portion Explorer, My Meals, Big Oven

Pantry List Notes, BugMe!, Notability

Refrigerator List Consume Within, Leftovers

Food Safety Food Safety at Home, USDA Food Safety (not produced by the USDA)

Grocery Shop Grocery Guru, Diabetes Fooducate, Grocery IQ, Smarter Shopping, iAteGreat, Seafood Watch, Smarter Shopping with Phil Lempert

Spices iSpice

Produce Fresh Fruit, Produce Guide, Food Focus: Fruits game, Veggie Garden Palooza game

Diabetes Drawer Glucagon

Organizations Diabetes Forecast (by ADA), Pocket First Aid & CPR (by AHA)

Check out these websites for more healthy shopping tips: www.supermarketsavvy.com and www.nuval.com.

they start to cook. Ingredients are already chopped and measured. Cookware and utensils ready to go. *Mise en place* makes meal preparation efficient and kitchen clean up a breeze.

- Plan out your meals for the next three days (or even the next week). Do you have all of the ingredients you need for your diabetes-friendly meals and snacks? Make sure that everything you need for your meals (including ingredients for recipes, cookware, measuring tools, and cutting boards) is easily accessible. Use the sheet that follows to help with your planning.
- Chop and dice veggies in advance and store them in labeled plastic bags in the refrigerator. That way you can simply toss them into your dish when you're ready to cook.
- Defrost meats and poultry a day or two prior to use. Make sure to defrost foods in the refrigerator and not on the counter.

Robin Plotkin, RD, LD, says, *"If cutting and chopping fresh fruits and vegetables is your downfall, Achilles heel, or whatever, purchase precut items from the produce department or from the salad bar. It's worth the extra money to ensure that you'll eat the fruits and veggies rather than watch them spoil and throw them away. Either way, you'll get more nutrition and likely save money in the long run."*

- Make several batches of healthy dishes, such as quinoa and beans, at one time so they are easy to use during the week. Or, cook large meals in your slow-cooker and freeze leftovers for quick dinners next week.

We asked Chef Robert Lewis, *The Happy Diabetic* and a person with type 2 diabetes, about his passion for cooking. When he was diagnosed with diabetes in 1998, Robert became motivated to create great-tasting dishes that were easy to prepare. Chef Robert says, *"Write down all the ingredients in your recipe before you go food shopping. Check off what you already have in the pantry, so you don't spend money on items you have in stock at home."* Great advice!

Meal Planning

Day 1

Breakfast _____

_____

Lunch _____

_____

Dinner _____

_____

Healthy Snacks _____

_____

Ingredients Needed

_____

_____

_____

_____

_____

_____

_____

_____

Day 2

Breakfast _____

_____

Lunch _____

_____

Dinner _____

_____

Healthy Snacks _____

_____

Ingredients Needed

_____

_____

_____

_____

_____

_____

_____

_____

Day 3

Breakfast _____

_____

Lunch _____

_____

Dinner _____

_____

Healthy Snacks _____

_____

Ingredients Needed

_____

_____

_____

_____

_____

_____

_____

_____

Visit www.sprypubdiabetes to download a printable pdf.

Meal preparation can be a challenge when you try to maintain a diabetes-friendly kitchen. How do you know what foods to purchase to prepare healthy meals? What are the best portable snacks to grab when on the go? What if you are a vegetarian? Kosher? Gluten-free? Lactose-intolerant? If you need serious guidance on meal planning and preparation, consider meeting with a registered dietitian-nutritionist who is also a certified diabetes educator. Together you can incorporate your food preferences into a healthy meal plan tailored specifically for your needs.

Diabetes-Friendly Recipes

Check out Chef Robert's delicious (and easy-breezy) recipes. These recipes are bound to be a hit for the entire family!

Chef Robert's Mediterranean Chicken of Love
Ingredients

Servings 4
Nutrition Facts
(per serving)
262 calories
23 g carbohydrates
6 g fat
33 g protein
8 g fiber

Recipe by Robert Lewis, www. happydiabetic.com

From the Produce Section
1 tomato, diced
3 fresh mushrooms
½ red pepper
½ green pepper
1 Tbsp chopped fresh parsley
¼ lime

From the Pantry
2 tsp extra virgin olive oil
¼ cup white wine or vegetable stock
1 Tbsp dried oregano
1 Tbsp jarred chopped garlic
1 can garbanzo beans drained and rinsed

1 Tbsp chopped dried basil
10 pitted black olives
Pepper to taste

From the Meat Market
1 pound skinless, boneless cooked chicken breast halves, sliced

Tools
1 12-inch nonstick skillet
1 wooden spoon
10-inch chef knife
1 cutting board

Directions

Heat oil in a large skillet over medium heat. Sauté all the vegetables and garlic for 3–5 minutes. Then add tomatoes and beans; sauté for 2–3 minutes. Lower heat, add white wine, and simmer for about 5 minutes. Add oregano, rosemary, and basil and simmer for 2–3 minutes more. Add the precooked chicken and simmer over low heat until chicken is completely heated through. Add olives and parsley to the skillet and cook for 1 minute. Season with pepper to taste and serve.

Happy Diabetic Shrimp Scampi

Shrimp and garlic go together like no other combination! This recipe makes a great appetizer or side dish. It's one of my favorites because it takes very little time to make. This is a twist on the classic scampi ... only much more HAPPY!

Ingredients

From the Produce Section
1 large tomato (4 slices)
4–5 sprigs of fresh basil
1 fresh lime

From the Dairy Section
2 oz. low-fat Feta cheese

From the Frozen Food Section
4 extra-large cooked shrimp

From the Pantry
Dash cracked pepper
2 tsp extra virgin olive oil
1 clove garlic, minced
¼ tsp freshly ground black pepper

Tools
10-inch serrated knife
1 large plate
9-inch nonstick sauté pan

Servings 4
Nutrition Facts
 (per serving)
68 calories
  1 g carbohydrates
  4 g fat
  7 g protein
0.5 g fiber

Recipe by Robert Lewis, www. happydiabetic.com

Directions

Wash and slice tomatoes crosswise into ½-inch-thick slices. Arrange 4 slices on a large salad plate. Sprinkle the Feta cheese on top of each tomato. Cut fresh basil leaves into strips and top sliced tomato with basil. Heat the olive oil in a pan and add the garlic and the shrimp. Cook until heated through. If you are using cooked shrimp, it should take about 3 minutes. (If you are using raw shrimp, it should take about 5–6 minutes.) Place the cooked shrimp on the tomatoes and drizzle the garlic and olive oil mixture over the cheese and shrimp. Add a dash of pepper and a squeeze of fresh lime. Enjoy!

Frozen Food vs. Scratch

We know that you are very busy. Do you ever have one of those days when you simply can't prepare a dinner meal and you don't have any leftovers? Keep a few healthy frozen meals on hand for an occasional quick meal. Here's what you should look for when selecting healthy frozen meal options.

- Choose a meal with a short list of ingredients. If the list is too long, or the ingredients are impossible to pronounce, the product probably contains too many preservatives and additives.
- Select frozen entrees that contain between 300 and 500 calories. Anything lower than 300 calories may leave you hungry afterward and make you more likely to reach for an unhealthy snack.
- Keep total fat to less than 30 percent and avoid all meals that contain trans fat. Be sure to check the ingredient label for the words *partially hydrogenated*. This is the code word for trans fat.
- Sodium (the mineral and main ingredient in table salt) should be no more than 200 mg for every 100 calories. For example, for a meal with 350 calories, select one that has 700 mg of sodium or less. Although it is not necessarily very low in sodium, it is your best choice. The United States Department of Agriculture and the American Heart Association recommend that people with or without diabetes should limit their sodium intake to 1,500 mg of sodium per day.
- Check the total carbohydrate, fiber, and sugar alcohol content of the product. Select entrees with at least 5 grams of fiber.

Avoid frozen entrees that contain prepared desserts.

- Always cook an extra side of vegetables. Most frozen entrees (even the advertised healthy ones) do not contain enough vegetables. Fresh is always best, but if you are pressed for time, microwave a frozen steamer bag. Fresh veggies are not only low in calories and high in fiber, but they also add color and crunch to your frozen meals. Keep cans of no-added-salt vegetables on hand in case fresh or frozen vegetables are not available.
- The American Heart Association has a Heart-Check mark for foods low in sodium, fat, saturated fat, trans fat, and cholesterol, but high in important vitamins and minerals. This symbol does not necessarily mean that a particular item is a "perfect choice," but it can help you make better selections.

Fill Up Your Diabetes–Friendly Pantry

Below is a list of products that would fit nicely into any pantry, including one belonging to a person with diabetes. See how many you can find in your pantry and then pick up a few on your next visit to the grocery store to try.

- ☐ Brown rice cakes
- ☐ Canned beans—black, garbanzo, lentils, pinto, red kidney
- ☐ Cooking oils—canola, extra virgin olive, grape seed
- ☐ Grains—barley, brown rice, couscous, oats, quinoa, whole-wheat pasta
- ☐ Low-sodium canned tomatoes, tomato sauce, tomato soup, broth-based vegetable soups
- ☐ Low-sodium vegetable juice
- ☐ Natural nut butters—almond butter and peanut butter
- ☐ Nonstick cooking sprays
- ☐ Oats and oatmeal (not instant)
- ☐ Popcorn (snack-size bags or kernels for air-popping)
- ☐ Reduced-sugar jams, jellies, and pancake syrups
- ☐ Snack and meal replacement bars
- ☐ Unsalted nuts—almonds, Brazil, pistachios, walnuts
- ☐ Vinegars—balsamic, red wine, white wine, rice, apple cider
- ☐ Water-packed canned chicken breast, salmon, sardines, and tuna
- ☐ 100% whole grain bread (containing at least 5 g fiber per serving)
- ☐ Whole grain cereals (containing at least 5 g fiber per serving)
- ☐ Whole grain crackers
- ☐ Whole wheat or nut flours—almond, coconut, or chickpea (some chefs suggest keeping nut flours in the freezer for a longer shelf life)
- ☐ Whole wheat pancake mix

Spice Up Your Diabetes-Friendly Kitchen

Hold the salt! Stock up on these spices to help perk up your taste buds and help improve your diabetes and cardiovascular health in the process.

- [ ] Basil
- [ ] Bay leaves
- [ ] Cayenne pepper
- [ ] Cinnamon
- [ ] Cumin
- [ ] Curry powder
- [ ] Garlic and onion powders (not onion or garlic salt)
- [ ] Ginger
- [ ] Helba (Fenugreek)
- [ ] Mrs. Dash, Mr. Dash
- [ ] Oregano
- [ ] Red pepper flakes
- [ ] Rosemary
- [ ] Salt-free spice rubs for meat and seafood
- [ ] Turmeric

Check expiration dates on the spice jars. It pays to try new spice combinations, too, to keep your healthy foods interesting.

Quick-Acting Carbohydrate Sources

Several sources of sugar or carbohydrates work well to treat low blood sugar (hypoglycemia), so keep them readily available. Treat hypoglycemia with a fast-acting source of carbohydrate such as fruit juices, hard candies, or glucose tablets. Foods that contain a high amount of fat as well as sugar and carbs, such as chocolate or cookies, do not work as quickly to raise blood sugar levels since fat slows the absorption of carbohydrates.

Discuss your target blood sugar range with your doctor. Together you will determine when to treat a low blood sugar level. Generally, if your blood glucose is below 70 mg/dL, one of these quick-fix foods should be consumed right away. Each of the following provides 15 grams of carbohydrate:

- ☐ ½ cup or 4 ounces of any 100% fruit juice
- ☐ 1 serving of glucose gel (the amount equal to 15 grams of carbohydrates)
- ☐ 3 to 4 glucose tablets (each tablet has about 3–4 grams of carbohydrate)
- ☐ 5 or 6 pieces of hard candy
- ☐ 1 tablespoon of honey or corn syrup
- ☐ 5 to 6 small Life Savers–type candies
- ☐ 3 to 5 peppermint hard candies
- ☐ 2 tablespoons of raisins
- ☐ 1 cup or 8 ounces of skim milk
- ☐ ½ cup or 4 ounces of a regular soft drink (not diet)

If your child has diabetes, create a healthy snack center. Designate one shelf, drawer, or spot on the kitchen counter for preportioned (carb-counted) go-to snacks. Have him or her help prepare the snack packages. This will allow your child to gain more independence and confidence when selecting a snack.

Notes _____

_____

_____

_____

_____

_____

_____

_____

_____

_____

_____

_____

_____

_____

_____

_____

_____

_____

Chapter Five

Get Up! Get Organized!

Setting Up a Morning Routine

Mornings can be hectic in any household. Add in blood glucose testing, insulin injections, or bolus corrections, and time becomes even more precious. Let's figure out how to better organize your morning routine because we know that having enough time to get everything done sets a positive tone for the day ahead.

The first step to facing your day with confidence is to create a checklist of what HAS to get done each morning. We suggest you write or type your list and keep it on your nightstand, post it to the bathroom mirror, or tack it on the refrigerator door. Post the checklist wherever you are going to see it as you get your morning going. If you see what needs to get accomplished each day, you are more likely to feel calm and be more productive.

One thing that you must do if you have diabetes is to check your blood sugar in the morning. While some parts of the morning routine can be shortened or changed, testing your blood sugar isn't one of them.

To quote Jeff Hitchcock, the founder of Children with Diabetes, *"The only bad blood sugar number is the one you don't know. If you have a child with type 1 diabetes, chances are that you might have checked his or her blood sugars several times during the night. Many adults with type 1 also check blood sugars overnight to make sure they are not running too low. In the morning, after testing blood sugars, the morning routine begins. If you usually take insulin and your blood sugar is running high, you might take your insulin before you begin your grooming routine."* Jeff's advice is spot on. Knowing your number before you get started in the morning is a "must-do."

Here's an example of a morning checklist. Don't get overwhelmed looking at this long list. Take a deep breath while you read over our suggested list and start to compile your own. We included a page for starting your personal list. Try to put everything in the order that works best for you.

Morning Checklist

- ☐ Check your blood sugar.
- ☐ Check your continuous glucose monitor (CGM), if you wear one.
- ☐ Meditate or stretch for a few minutes.
- ☐ Take your insulin and medications (timed correctly, of course).
- ☐ Fuel up! Prepare and eat breakfast.
- ☐ Take your vitamins or supplements as needed.
- ☐ Attend to children/spouse/elderly parents' needs.
- ☐ Feed/walk/attend to pets.
- ☐ Brush teeth.
- ☐ Shower (If time is at a premium, plan to shower the night before.)
- ☐ Grooming (shaving, styling hair, makeup application, etc.)
- ☐ Get dressed. Pick out your clothes the night before to streamline your morning routine.
- ☐ Finish preparing snacks and lunches. Pack up food for the day.
- ☐ Double check on diabetes supplies for the day.
- ☐ Make beds/unload dishwasher/tidy house.

My Morning Checklist

Every Day
- ☐ _____
- ☐ _____
- ☐ _____
- ☐ _____
- ☐ _____
- ☐ _____
- ☐ _____
- ☐ _____
- ☐ _____

This Morning
- ☐ _____
- ☐ _____
- ☐ _____
- ☐ _____
- ☐ _____
- ☐ _____
- ☐ _____
- ☐ _____
- ☐ _____

Appointments/Tasks for Today
- ☐ _____
- ☐ _____
- ☐ _____
- ☐ _____
- ☐ _____
- ☐ _____
- ☐ _____
- ☐ _____
- ☐ _____

Visit www.sprypubdiabetes to download a printable pdf.

Preparing the Night Before

Want to make the most of your morning? Have a well-thought-out plan in place before you get out of bed. A smooth morning is usually the result of proper planning and preparation, and that begins the night before.

Try to do a little prep work the night before and get a jump on the busy day ahead. Of course, if you are an early riser, then these tasks can be performed in the morning as well. Here's a list of possible evening "Can-Dos" to set you on the right track.

Lay out your clothes for the next day. Do the same for young children. This includes everything from accessories, undergarments, shoes, and coats. This is a HUGE time saver! Trust us!

Decide what you want for breakfast and get it ready. Set the coffee or tea pot for your morning brew. Get out utensils. Dispense oral medications and supplements or vitamins. Hard boil eggs and premeasure your oatmeal and almonds. You will shave minutes off your morning if you have breakfast ready to go the evening before.

Pack lunches and snacks. You might save a lot of time if you purchase individual servings of healthy ingredients, such as apple slices, nuts, hummus, string cheese, carrots, etc. If this is not economical for you, spend time on the weekends presorting these items into individual containers. Store perishable items in the refrigerator to keep them fresh. Lunch and snacks should be ready for morning grab-and-go.

Stock your diabetes supply bag. Make sure testing supplies and all necessary medications are at the ready. Insulin can easily go from refrigerator to tote in the morning. Don't forget a water bottle. A fun water bottle will remind you to hydrate throughout the day.

We asked the fabulous Max "Mr. Divabetic" Szadek (whose motto is "glam more, fear less") to share tips on how to glam up your morning routine. Max was the former long-time assistant to the remarkable Luther Vandross. He is the founder and creator of Divabetic. Max currently hosts Diva Talk Radio, which is a truly empowering and educational program. Max says, *"Don't be afraid to add some bling to your self-care routine. A daily dose of dazzle can be inspiring as well as easy. Bedazzle glucose testing supplies like your blood glucose monitor. Buy a fabulous looking water bottle or make an ordinary one look extraordinary. Oriental Trading Company has literally thousands of quick fix rhinestones and stickers you can add to a plain water bottle if you don't want to spend too much money. Purchase a bottle similar to your favorite sports star. You'll feel as fierce as Serena or Venus Williams when you drink out of a Nike water bottle. I recommend buying a water bottle for every bag, too. This way, you're never going thirsty."*

Prepack backpacks, purses, tote bags, gym bags, and briefcases, and place them in your home's "launching pad." A launching pad is one place in your home to corral all the items each family member must have before he or she leaves the house. An example of a launching pad could be next to your front door, at the entrance to your garage, or the house entrance or exit most used.

Make a reminder checklist for you and your family so no one forgets anything. List items such as cell phones, keys, wallets, lunch boxes and snack bags, homework, musical instruments, sporting equipment, diabetes supplies, etc. Tack it to a cork board or write it directly on a wipe board to make changes a breeze. Make sure to hang it right by the launching pad for all to see.

"Clean Sweep" your home. Tidy kitchen. Empty garbage. Run the dishwasher at night and unload in the morning (if time permits). Toss in laundry or fold and put away clean clothes. These tasks are time robbers during the morning rush, so set aside time the night before to complete household tasks.

Shower the night before. Have young children do the same. This cuts down on morning prep time significantly.

Set up a water schedule. If your goal is to drink 48 to 64 ounces of water a day, then plan your water breaks. For example, drink 8 ounces by 10 a.m., again by 1 p.m., etc. If you are not naturally thirsty, purposely schedule your water intake. You will stay well hydrated through the day.

Extra bonus? A soothing bath will help you calm down and unwind after the day. If showering in the morning is a "must-do" and wakes you up, limit your shower time to 10 minutes.

Create your roadmap for tomorrow. Go over your appointments and "to-dos" for the next day. A little bit of night time prep will pay off big time in the morning.

Good Morning Sunshine

Getting up in the morning is not easy for most. Who wants to leave the warmth of a cozy bed? But for those with diabetes getting up in the morning presents its own set of challenges. With a few strategies in place, hopefully getting going in the morning will be as stress free as possible.

We asked dancer, actress, and founder of Myabetic, Kyrra Richards how she gets her gorgeous self ready every morning and she shared some great tips with us. Kyrra says, *"Growing up dancing, I relied on muscle memory to remember my routines. I would practice the movement so much that the sequence became automatic. I could resist nerves and onstage distractions because my performance was so well rehearsed. This concept also applies to the choreography of my everyday life. At the sound of my morning alarm clock, it's showtime — wash my face, brush my teeth, apply*

SPF moisturizer, check my blood sugar (and correct with insulin if necessary), get dressed (often directly into workout attire so I don't have time to think of an excuse to avoid an early exercise session), hair/makeup, pack my bags (including my daily diabetes supplies), and go!

"After my diagnosis, I'll admit it took a while to integrate my diabetes chores into the routine. I would let hours go by before remembering to check my blood sugar and even forgot my meter, insulin, and supplies at home. I had to change my system and relearn the new method, just like when I was a little girl first learning my 'big girl' responsibilities. Instead of packing my fun, pink lunchbox with a thermos and baggies of snacks, I now pack my fun, pink diabetes wallet (because some things don't change) and refill its compartments with lancets, test strips, and other diabetes goodies.

"Diabetes is now part of your daily routine, but you can still make it your own. Organize in style! I didn't want to become a bag lady, lugging around suitcases of medical paraphernalia. Instead, I created a fashionable diabetes accessory company (Myabetic www.myabetic.com) that offers products specifically designed to help manage a healthy lifestyle." Kyrra is able to maintain her workouts, grooming routine, blood glucose testing, and insulin regime because she plans ahead.

Apps for Morning

Topic	iPhone	Android
Wake up	Clock, World Clock	World Clock & Widget, Clocks Around the World
Sleep	Fitbit	Fitbit
Pack Lunch	Pack Lunch Maker, Snack Wheel	
Water	8 Glasses a Day, Water Logged	
To Do	Reminders, Sticky Notes	
Music	iTunes, Pandora	Pandora
Blood Sugar	IBGStar, Vree	
Vitamins	Vitamin Tracker, Vitamate	Vitamin Tracker
Weight	Withings	FitScales

Source: Adapted from *An App A Day* and *An App A Day for Health Professionals*, © 2012, Frederico Arts LLC.

Tips to Help You Get Up and Go

Set an alarm. Avoid setting your clock to music if you have trouble getting up in the morning. Music tends to become white noise and lulls you back to sleep. Invest in multiple alarm clocks and place them around your room. This will automatically force you to get out of bed to turn them off.

Hit the ground running. Literally! Work with your energy cycle. For example, if exercising is important to you and you wake up each day ready to get your adrenaline going, then work out first thing in the morning when you are most motivated and more inclined to commit. Being refreshed and ready to go will help you move through your morning routine with ease.

Time your tasks. A common mistake people make in creating their morning schedules is being unrealistic about how long certain tasks take. To improve your morning routine, keep a time log for about a week or two noting how long each task takes you to accomplish. This information will help you plan your mornings better and establish how much time you actually need in the morning to get out the door stress free.

Beat the clock. Do you dawdle in the morning? Try "bill boarding." First, place an analog clock in each room of the house that you use in the morning. Make sure it is an analog clock so you can see the "sweep" of time. Hang a wipe board or giant post-it note next to the clock with the time you need to be OUT of that room written down. So for example, if you need to be out of the bathroom at 7:30 a.m. then post that on the board. Seeing time move alongside what time you need to be moving to the next activity will help motivate you and keep you on track.

Set it to music. Listening to music can invigorate your morning routine. Sound affects our mood and body. So if you need an energy boost to get going in the morning, don't be afraid to blast that old time rock 'n' roll to get yourself moving. If soothing music helps set the tone for the day, then have classical music playing while you move through your morning routine.

Ready. Set. Go! If you linger too long in bed or take a long time to eat breakfast, set a timer to keep everything and everyone on track. Our favorite? Time Timer (www.timetimer.com). The small red dial allows you to see the "sweep" of time passing.

Leave the House Organized

Your morning is now organized, so it's time to prepare to leave the house with confidence. You can tackle any curveball that might be thrown your way. We know you can!

What better way to be prepared for the day than to carry your supplies in a carryall or tote designated just for your diabetes supplies? A special diabetes "carrier" is not necessary. You can easily use any small backpack or tote bag just as long as your supplies are safe, handy, and organized. If you want a tote that is specifically designed for your diabetes supplies, check out some of our favorites:

Skidaddle Bags (www.skidaddlebags.com) Created by a mom whose child has type 1 diabetes, Skidaddle bags are fun and

Keep glucose tablets or some other fast-acting source of carbohydrate on your nightstand or next to your bed in case of a low blood sugar during the night or when you wake up. Don't keep super-sweet snacks at your fingertips. You might reach for them too often! Have you ever eaten a high-carbohydrate snack just before bed or in the middle of the night because it was nearby? You'll think twice if it isn't in easy reach.

fashionable. Designed with kids in mind, there are many bright colors and fun patterns from which to choose.

Betic Bag (www.beticbag.net) These bags are fun, fashionable, and functional all in one. Big and roomy with plenty of space for all your diabetes supplies.

The Insulin Case Shop (www.insulincase.com) This website is your one-stop shopping for all things diabetes. From medication lock boxes to pill organizers to handy travel cases, they have it all.

aDorn Designs (www.adorndesigns.com) Is it a handbag? A diabetes carryall? It's both. These handbags include a main compartment for all your day-to-day stuff AND a separate zip-out removable clutch to hold all your supplies.

Avon's Butler Organizer Tote Bag (www.avon.com) Although it is not designed specifically for diabetes supplies, this tote is the world's first compartmentalized bag. The totes contain built-in organizing slots for all your day-to-day essentials.

The Diabetes Readi Pak (www.readionthego.com) Designed by Sanofi, it has a large insulated main compartment, two mesh side pockets (for water bottles), and a zippered back compartment.

> Keep an index card pinned to your supply bag to ensure that everything that should be in the bag IS! Place a list of medications, medical contact information, and your cell phone contact information in the bag in case it gets lost or misplaced.

Myabetic bags and accessories (www.myabetic.com) It's time for a diabetes makeover! These accessories for men, women, and children come in fun, fashionable colors and fabrics. Myabetic's supply wallets, kits, handbags, and device-specific cases accommodate everyday diabetes needs with specific compartments, pockets, elastic loops, and removable waste pouches. Manage your health in style and celebrate your individuality.

More from Max, Mr. Divabetic, *"A little sparkle can go a long way and keep you motivated. Buy a cute small pouch for your supplies. Choose colors or patterns that make you smile. You use it every day so it should be FABULOUS! Throw in a few nail stickers and a nail file in your bag, too. This way, if you're treating a low blood sugar on the go by following the Rule of 15 you can give yourself a quick, fun, safe manicure. And stickers make it easy! Plus, if you make mistakes you can just peel it off. Get sexy! Cut out a picture of your favorite celebrity 'sugar substitute' and put him in your bag. Bradley Cooper, George Clooney, Usher, and Tatum Channing smiling at you while you're taking your blood glucose can make the experience more enjoyable."*

It's All in the Bag

Here are our suggestions for some of the things needed in your bag.

- ☐ Insulin (if needed)
- ☐ Medications (in measured doses)
- ☐ Glucose meter and testing supplies
- ☐ Fast-acting source of glucose/carbohydrate (such as glucose tablets or glucose gel)
- ☐ Nonperishable healthy snacks (such as unsalted nuts, dried fruit, peanut butter on whole grain crackers, or healthy high-fiber granola bars)
- ☐ Lunch or other meals (in an insulated bag)
- ☐ Water bottle
- ☐ Contact information (including emergency contacts and medical information)
- ☐ Emergency phone numbers
- ☐ Cell phone and charger
- ☐ Non-nutritive or artificial sweeteners (in case your favorite is not available when eating out)
- ☐ _____
- ☐ _____
- ☐ _____
- ☐ _____
- ☐ _____
- ☐ _____
- ☐ _____
- ☐ _____
- ☐ _____
- ☐ _____
- ☐ _____
- ☐ _____
- ☐ _____

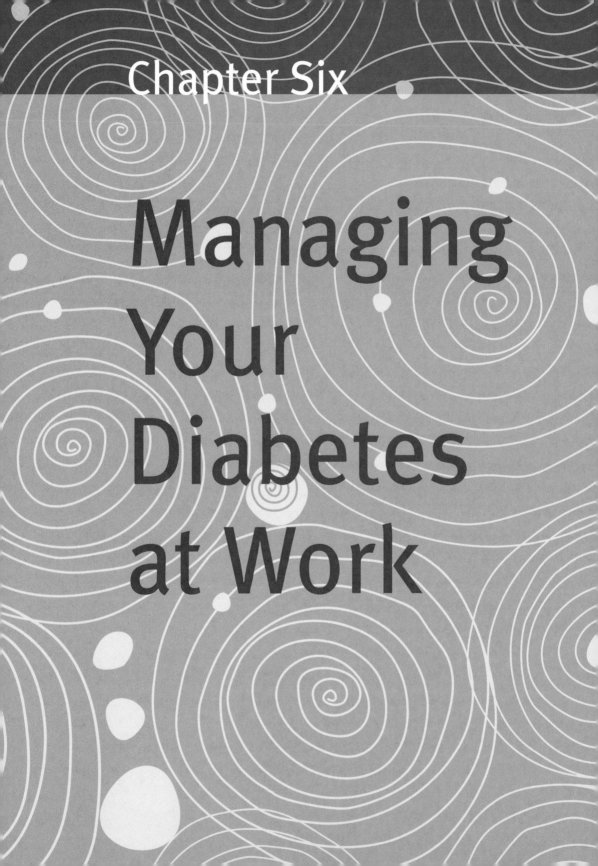

Chapter Six

Managing Your Diabetes at Work

HAVE YOU EVER READ SOMETHING at work (or at home) three times because the words just didn't seem to make sense? At some point, you probably realized that you worked straight through lunch. Your blood sugar might have dropped because you didn't eat for a long period of time and, as a result, you lost your ability to focus. Finally, you tested your blood sugar and realized that your lack of focus was due to a low blood sugar level. Once you started to eat foods that contained carbohydrates (or took a blood glucose tablet or a swig of juice), your blood sugar probably climbed into a more acceptable range. You were able to focus on what you were trying to read and the world around you started to make more sense. Does that scenario sound familiar? Do you experience these types of hypoglycemic episodes at work? Whether you work in an office, as a teacher, or outside in construction, we can help you stay organized so that you can hopefully keep your diabetes under control. If you improve your diabetes management, you can start to significantly increase your productivity at your job. No worries! Help is on the way. Here are some tips and tricks on how to keep your diabetes organized at work.

Map Out Your Schedule

Take some time today to think about how your workdays and weekends tend to unfold. Are you one of those people with a very regular (or predictable) schedule? For example, do you take the same train each morning and evening, or leave your house to drive to work at the same time every day? Do you have regular meetings or appointments and generally eat lunch around the same time? Do you leave your office, school, or work site at the same time most days? Or do you have many days that are completely unpredictable or work rotating shifts? Do you travel very often for business? Once you understand how your workdays progress, it's important to establish set times to test your blood sugar and take your insulin or medications. You can also figure out the best times for eating meals and snacks throughout your workday.

If your workdays are predictable, these times will be fairly repetitive, meaning the time you test your blood sugars will likely be about the same times every day. If your workdays vary, it will take a bit more effort to determine the best times for you to test your blood sugar, take your medications or insulin, and eat. The easiest way to organize this is to plan *in advance* and determine those times as best you can.

- When possible, try to eat your breakfast, lunch, and snacks around the same time every day. This can help you properly manage your diabetes, as well as serve as a reminder to eat. Skipping meals and snacks is a recipe for a hypoglycemic disaster at work.
- Please don't treat your diabetes as something you can manage on the fly. You can help to prevent problems at work (such as a hypoglycemic episode at a critical time) if you know your blood sugar number, so test and eat as planned. Of course, you'll also feel better and might even prevent complications due to poorly controlled blood sugar levels in the long run.

We asked Scott Herman, Executive Vice President of Operations/CBS Radio and person with type 2 diabetes about how he manages his diabetes during his hectic workday.

Scott says, *"I am a creature of habit and because I'm on the road virtually three weeks a month I find it's easier for me to keep to my normal schedule and routine when it comes to testing and meds. Just as I have meetings and appointments scheduled throughout the day (and sometimes evenings), I test my blood sugars on-time, several times every day. I can't afford to lose focus during an important meeting, especially when I'm traveling across time zones.*

"I always test my fasting blood sugar right after I get dressed and just before I leave to start my day. I test before lunch even though my number is very consistent. I also test my evening blood sugar because I often eat out in restaurants, which might affect my numbers. It's important for me not to leave anything to chance. Aside from that, I also test when I'm feeling funny. After so many years of dealing with diabetes, I know my body ... I know when my sugar is high (fuzzy vision) or when it's low (lethargic and tired). But I'm a numbers guy, so I test my blood sugars often and treat a high or low blood sugar as needed.

"I take my Victoza injection when I'm getting dressed in the morning and my insulin injection when I'm getting ready for bed at night. Oral meds are taken with breakfast and dinner. This routine helps me prevent a missed dosage. I always fill my weekly pill boxes on Sundays so I know that I have a full week's worth with me and I always take enough medicine to last me three extra days in case I get stuck in a city due to weather or plane issues. I'm always prepared whether I'm in the office in NYC or at a meeting in LA ... and everywhere in-between!"

Treat Your Diabetes-Related Activities as Appointments

Once you've mapped out your workdays and figured out the best times to test your blood sugar and eat, input those times into your calendar as appointments. It doesn't matter if you use a written schedule book, a calendar on your computer, and/or smartphone, or have an assistant who handles your schedule. Always include your diabetes-related activities in your daily calendar to serve as a reminder. And, as the rest of your schedule starts to take shape with meetings and appointments, you'll already have time set aside to properly manage your diabetes.

For example, let's say that your calendar has an entry to check your blood glucose at 11:00 a.m. If your boss asks you to participate in a conference call at 11:00 a.m., you will see the "Check Blood Sugar" entry and be reminded to make sure you check your blood before the call. Think about the same situation where you hadn't entered the time to check your blood sugar. Your calendar shows a conference call at 11:00 a.m., for which you have to get ready. Your morning is ridiculously busy, but you get everything finished for the call and then dial in. The call runs over an hour and toward the end you are spacing out and missing parts of the discussion. Just then, you realize you never checked your blood the hour before as you usually would have done. Had the blood sugar check been on your calendar, you probably would have included that as one of the things to get finished before the call and you would have avoided the hypoglycemic episode.

We asked Dr. Beverly Adler (author, clinical psychologist, certified diabetes educator, and PWD) about how she handles her busy workday. Dr. Bev says, *"I specialize in treating the emotional issues of patients with diabetes in my private practice. I not only discuss issues of adjustment to being diagnosed with diabetes, but I also consider myself to be a role model to others who live with diabetes. And keeping it together during a long workday can be quite challenging! I have had type 1 diabetes for 38 years (with no complications). So keeping my office diabetes friendly helps not only me but my patients, as well. I keep small boxes of juice in the office as well as glucose tablets for me and my patients, in case we need a fast acting source of glucose. I have shared my supplies on many occasions. Sometimes, my schedule gets very hectic and I need a quick snack to tide me over until my next meal. I keep "chewy bars" (with 10 grams of protein) in my drawer for a quick snack. I also keep almonds in my desk to munch on between appointments. Ironically, I have lollipops available in the office for blood sugar lows—which many patients without diabetes also enjoy!*

"I regularly check my blood sugar during the day. I try to check between appointments, but if I am in session and I feel like my blood sugar is dropping, I will check in front of my patient. I use it as a teachable moment to "Test! Don't guess!" as they say on www.dLife.com (a website devoted to diabetes).

"I also try to stay hydrated during the day. I generally keep a bottled beverage on my desk and take small sips throughout the day. One day I was drinking from a water bottle that was filled with an orange liquid. Since my patient knew I had juice in the office for emergencies, she became alarmed and thought I was treating a hypoglycemic reaction with orange juice. I reassured her that it was only a zero calorie orange flavor packet that I had added to the water. It was nice to know that my patients care as much about me as I do about them."

Your Most Important Customer

Based on the type of work that you do, you might have certain customers or clients or accounts that take priority over others. These are the ones that are so important that, when they are scheduled, you make every effort to stick to the schedule and not cancel. Your diabetes-related activities need to be treated the same way. Once they are scheduled, you should make every effort to keep them where they are and not move them around too much. If you do have to make some time adjustments, just remember that YOU and YOUR HEALTH must be a priority. So don't blow it off!

Build Buffer Time around Your Activities

While it is sometimes difficult, try not to stack a meeting and appointments on top of one another. Invariably, things run over and schedules get out of whack. And that makes tackling your diabetes-related activities, even those in your calendar, that much harder. Try to leave gaps of time between items in your calendar, which will serve as natural pressure relief valves and help you accomplish all of your tasks.

- Let's say you are scheduled to meet with a colleague to discuss a presentation on a particular day at 11:00 a.m., and you are aware that you have a repeat appointment reminder in your calendar to test your blood sugar every day at 12:00 noon. In addition, you have another meeting with a potential client at 12:30 p.m. We've all had days like that! Try to make sure that your first meeting ends no later than 11:50 a.m. That

10-minute gap should give you enough time to test your blood sugar and treat a low if necessary. If your blood sugar is low, re-test in another 15 minutes and treat again if necessary. Now you can catch up on things before your next appointment and eat a quick lunch, too.

Move Around and Stay Active

Stay active during your workday. By being physically active, you can help to improve your blood sugar levels and hopefully gain more mental focus. If you have a sedentary job, move your feet up and down and around while you're sitting at your desk. Try to walk up and down the staircase or around your office floor a few times a day. Find a buddy and take a walk after you eat your lunch or during break-time. Keep some light weights or Pilates bands underneath your desk and lift them over your head every so often for a nice stretch. You'll keep your arms toned and burn a few calories at the same time. Reach for a weight under your desk rather than a cookie in the office pantry. What a great way to stay healthy and avoid extra calories, carbs, salt, and fat!

Keeping Diabetes Supplies Organized at Work

Now that you have your workday schedule in place, it's time to think about how to organize your diabetes supplies at work. After all, it's good to have an appointment reminder to check your blood sugar at 3:00 every afternoon, but what if your meter and testing supplies are nowhere to be found? Here's what we suggest you do to manage your supplies:

- **Designate a supply drawer, box, or shelf in your work area.**
  Whether you work at a desk, behind a cash register, or on a
  construction site, designate a space that is *solely* for your
  diabetes supplies, such as your meter, solutions, test strips,
  lancets, fast-acting glucose (or tablets), syringes, and medications
  or insulin (in a cool place or refrigerator). Since you spend almost
  as much time at work as you do at home (sometimes even more),
  this supply cache should be as complete and comprehensive as
  the one you have at home. Designate a single spot for your
  supplies, and make sure your supplies are completely stocked.
  Then, you won't have to search for a test strip when you are in
  the middle of a hectic day.
- **Tell your coworkers and colleagues about your supplies.** Imagine
  this, you get called down the hall for an urgent meeting. You're
  stuck in a conference room when your blood sugar level starts to
  plummet. However, your glucose tablets and your juice box are
  sitting in your supply drawer at your desk. Would you want to have
  to spend the time to explain to your assistant or colleagues how
  to find your supplies or what the glucose tablet container looks
  like? Of course not. Tell your coworkers about your supplies and
  how they can help you if you become hypoglycemic. If you need
  them, they will know how to help. Share some of this basic
  information at work. You know that a few precious seconds could
  be the difference between a minor speed bump in your day and a
  major health problem at work.
- **Create a portable "work only" supply kit.** In addition to a supply

kit at work, create one for your daily commute. You can also use this portable kit for an important meeting or appointment outside your office or workplace. If you carry a briefcase, knapsack, or bag with compartments, designate one of those for your "must-have" diabetes-related supplies. If you carry a tote or similar bag, keep your supplies in a self-contained smaller bag. In order to help ensure that this supply kit is always stocked, you should inventory and restock it regularly.

Take a few minutes on Sunday evening to restock your diabetes supply bag. If you work on the weekends, restock your supply bag after a day off. You'll be refreshed and able to better assess your inventory for the week ahead. Set a reminder on your smartphone calendar to restock your diabetes supply bag.

Work Challenges

We've given you several strategies for people with diabetes to use at work, but it pays to spend a few minutes thinking about any individual challenges you have faced at work in dealing with your diabetes. Next, consider possible ways to change something in your surroundings to improve the situation. If you get stuck on a solution, don't hesitate to discuss the challenge with your supervisor or coworkers.

Challenge 1 _____

Possible Resolutions _____

_____

_____

_____

Challenge 2 _____

Possible Resolutions _____

_____

_____

_____

Challenge 3 _____

Possible Resolutions _____

_____

_____

_____

Challenge 4 _____

Possible Resolutions _____

_____

_____

_____

Notes _____

Chapter Seven

End the Day the Healthy Diabetes Way

WHEW! YOU'RE FINALLY HOME AND NOW it's time to start the second part of your day. Just like Act Two of a Broadway play. We want to help you accomplish your evening activities with the same positive attitude you used to tackle your morning routine. Whether you are a stay-at-home mom or dad, a corporate executive, or a police officer, time moves quickly, especially when the sun starts to set. Add in blood sugar testing, meal preparation, family obligations, medications and insulin adjustments, and every minute becomes precious. Let's work together to better organize your evening routine and help you accomplish your goals. Wouldn't it be nice to have a restful and relaxing evening? We think so, too. Let's get started.

An Essential Checklist

The first step is to create a checklist of what HAS to get done each night. We suggest you begin to write down your evening to-do list. See what needs to get accomplished each evening and then check off each item as you complete the task on the list. You can actually follow your progress and stay motivated. Soon you're likely to feel more calm and productive.

Here are some examples of what might belong on your evening checklist. Don't get overwhelmed when you initially look at this long list. Please remember that these are just suggestions. You can use them to help you create a list that works for you! Remember to organize the list in an order that works best for you.

Evening Checklist

- [ ] Take your medications and insulin as prescribed
- [ ] Prepare and cook a nutritious dinner
- [ ] Clean up the kitchen after dinner
- [ ] Test your blood sugar before dinner and before bedtime (or as suggested by your doctor)
- [ ] Tend to elderly parents' needs
- [ ] Prepare breakfast, lunch, and snacks for the next day (foods that can be prepared in advance)
- [ ] Put together diabetes supplies for the following day
- [ ] Set up medications for the week or next day
- [ ] Tidy house/laundry
- [ ] Exercise (if part of your routine)
- [ ] Check mail, pay bills, return phone calls
- [ ] Tend to pets' needs
- [ ] Help children with homework or other activities
- [ ] Shower and groom (as needed)
- [ ] Lay out your clothes and your children's clothes for the next day
- [ ] Check your calendar for the next day's schedule

Now think about your evening routine and create a reminder checklist of your to-do items.

My Evening Checklist

Every Day

☐ _____
☐ _____
☐ _____
☐ _____
☐ _____
☐ _____

This Evening

☐ _____
☐ _____
☐ _____
☐ _____
☐ _____
☐ _____

Appointments/Tasks for Tomorrow

☐ _____
☐ _____
☐ _____
☐ _____
☐ _____
☐ _____

Some evenings you may need to attend a meeting, drive children to various events, return important phone calls, and go through your mail. Maybe your commute didn't go as planned and you have less time to get through all of your evening tasks. You might even have planned a much-needed night out with friends. You probably realize that not every day is exactly the same, and, therefore, it's important to be flexible. Just remember that if you have a basic routine in place, you're more likely to feel in control of your evening. Try to follow some of the guidelines in this chapter. Soon you may feel less overwhelmed and will become more accomplished.

Organize Your Meal Schedule

In chapter 4, we describe a step-by-step approach to organizing your refrigerator, pantry, and freezer. We also give you tips and tools on how to grocery shop more efficiently. Once you have all of your cooking supplies organized in your kitchen, you can create a meal schedule for the week. A weekly meal schedule can help you make healthy choices that may help you control your blood sugar levels. You'll also be more likely to manage your weight. Best of all, you won't come home and feel anxious and worry about what's for dinner.

Take Inventory of Your Food

Once you follow the steps outlined in the kitchen chapters, you'll have a well-stocked and organized refrigerator, freezer, and pantry. Make sure that you have all of the basic foods and ingredients you might need to plan healthy and well-balanced meals for the week ahead. Keep a written list of any basic items you will need to purchase for the following week.

Plan and Write Down Your Meals for the Week Ahead

Refer to the Meal Planning chart, page 78. Are there food items that weren't used last week? Try and include those ingredients in a recipe this week. Check out some healthy, diabetes-friendly cookbooks from your local library or look online at www.cookinglight.com, www.dLife.com, or www.diabeteseveryday.com or ideas on simple and healthy recipes that are within your calorie, carbohydrate, and fat budgets. If possible, meet with a registered dietitian-nutritionist who is also a certified diabetes educator. He or she can help you develop a healthy meal plan that includes some of your favorite foods. You can eat well, control your blood sugar levels, and enjoy what you eat.

Keep a simple written plan of your meals for the week ahead. You are more likely to eat nutritious and properly portioned meals if you generally stay within your preplanned menu guidelines. Of course, you don't have to always plan exactly what you are going to eat. However, if you leave your meals up to chance, you might consume more fast food or take-out. Try to cook more of your own meals so that you know what ingredients are used and have more control over your health and blood sugar levels.

Prepare to Go Shopping

You've chosen your meals and may have included any leftovers from last week. Using the current menu plan and recipes, check the pantry, refrigerator, and freezer for the necessary items and add to your initial grocery list of basic items. Don't forget to take the coupons!

Are You Really Hungry?

Before you eat, think about how hungry you are on the scale below. Select a "0" if you are so hungry that you can't think straight and might have a low blood sugar. Select a "5" if you are so stuffed that you need to unbutton your pants. Hopefully, you won't be at the extreme ends of the scale too often. Use this scale as a tool to help you decide if you are hungry or if you want to eat for another reason (such as stress or boredom). Test your blood sugar, especially if you are at the high or low end of the scale. Remember, there is no right or wrong answer.

	0	1	2	3	4	5

0   I am starving. It's hard to think and I feel dizzy. I will test my blood sugar and eat.

1   I am very hungry. I will test my blood sugar before I eat.

2   I am hungry. I look forward to my next meal or snack. I might have to eat earlier than usual, after I test my blood sugar.

3   I am satisfied. I feel comfortable and satisfied after my last meal or snack.

4   I am full because I overate. I feel uncomfortable and will test my blood sugar.

5   I am overstuffed and need to unbutton my pants. I will test my blood sugar.

Use a Slow Cooker

Try using a slow cooker. Follow each step in the recipe to help ensure that you use adequate liquids and seasonings. Put the ingredients in the cooker, set the time, and get on with the rest of your activities. You can cook healthy, well-balanced meals, including lean protein (such as chicken, turkey, or lean pork) along with vegetables in a slow cooker. You'll have a one-pot meal that's truly enjoyable.

> Use a slow cooker liner to make clean-up a snap.

Chop and Dice in Advance

Try to do as much advance food prep work for the following day in the evening as you clean up the kitchen. If tomorrow night's dinner requires chopped celery, onions, and cubed chicken, make sure that it's all ready to go the night before. Store raw meat, poultry, and sea-food in separate containers or tightly sealed, labeled storage bags. Remember to always place raw protein

> Remember to keep extra cut and washed veggies on hand in case you need a crunchy snack while you are in the midst of preparation. Low-calorie, high-fiber vegetables make a great anytime snack that shouldn't have a signifi-cant effect on your blood sugar level.

foods on the bottom shelf in the refrigerator in case anything drips from the package. By following these rules, you'll be sure to limit bacterial issues and avoid cross contamination. Once you start to prepare your meal for the following evening, you'll have everything ready to go.

Prepare Enough of Your Favorite Dish for Four Nights

Freeze two portions and serve the other two on alternate nights. For example, you can have one serving on Monday and the other on Wednesday evening. The following week you can defrost your delicious creation on Tuesday and Thursday nights for dinner. Make sure to clearly mark all freezer foods with the name of the dish and the date of preparation.

Food Journal

Use a food journal to write down your meal plan in black ink. Chances are that you might make some changes as the week progresses. No worries! It's good to listen to your body and make changes based on your level of hunger and physical activity. Next, write down what you actually ate in red ink. That way you can keep track of what you eat and tweak future menus to better fit your needs. Doesn't that sound like a great plan?

Every evening, make sure you review your meal plan for the next day. If you need to buy fresh produce for a particular meal or recipe, make sure that you or another member of your household is able to pick it up. Plan a quick trip to the supermarket or local green grocer prior to meal preparation time. Otherwise, you might miss an ingredient or two for your recipe.

Daily Diabetes Blood Sugar, Hunger, Food, Exercise, and Water Log

(Record your blood sugars, hunger scale number, what you eat for each meal and snack, exercise details (type and duration), and each 8 oz. of water (with a ✓).

Date _____

Exercise	
Water	
Blood sugar	
Hunger scale	
Breakfast	
Blood sugar	
Hunger scale	
Morning snack	
Blood sugar	
Hunger scale	
Lunch	
Blood sugar	
Hunger scale	
Afternoon snack	
Blood sugar	
Hunger scale	
Dinner	
Blood sugar	
Hunger scale	
Evening snack	
Notes	

Tackling Tomorrow's To-Dos

What can you do in the evening to make tomorrow morning easier? Have a well-thought-out plan in place before you go to bed! You see, a smooth morning begins the night before. Of course if you are an early riser, then these tasks can be performed in the morning as well. As we said in our morning chapter, we can't stress enough how important it is to get organized the night before to ensure an easy morning. Figure out what works best for you at any time of day. We'll remind you of some of the possible evening "can-dos" to start tomorrow morning off right.

Lay out all your clothes for the next day. Do the same for young children. This includes everything from accessories, undergarments, shoes, and coats. This is a HUGE time saver. Trust us!

Decide what you want for breakfast and get it ready. Set the coffee or tea pot for your morning brew. Get out utensils. Dispense oral medications, supplements, or vitamins. Hard boil eggs and premeasure your oatmeal and almonds. You will shave minutes off your morning if you have breakfast ready to go the evening before.

Pack lunches and snacks. Consider purchasing individual servings of healthy ingredients such as apple slices, nuts, hummus, string cheese, carrots, etc. If this is not economical for you, spend time on the weekends presorting these items into individual containers. Store perishable items in the refrigerator to keep them fresh. Lunch and snacks should be ready for morning grab-and-go.

We asked author Gary Scheiner, MS, CDE, PWD, and 2013 AADE Diabetes Educator of the Year, about his blood sugar testing during his evening routine. Gary says, *"It is more important to check BG at bedtime than at any other time of day. Knowing where you are allows you to fix what might be off. If you're above target, a correction dose of insulin (conservative in most cases) will keep you from running high through the night and ruining a good night's sleep, not to mention your A1c. If you're a little on the low side before bed, a modest snack can return you to a safe range and help avoid a dangerous middle-of-the-night low. Better yet, if you're wearing a CGM, take the direction of your BG into account as well. A normal BG that is dropping quickly will require a different response than one that is stable or rising. Bottom line: knowing your BG status at bedtime lets you make smart decisions and enjoy a good night's sleep. If you've had a high-fat meal (like a restaurant meal) at dinnertime, a normal BG at bedtime can be misleading. You'll probably rise through the night due to the effects of the dietary fat. If you want to avoid morning highs after high-fat meals the night before, talk to your doctor or diabetes educator about increasing your basal insulin or taking a small dose of NPH insulin at bedtime."*

Stock your diabetes supply bag. Make sure testing supplies and all necessary medications are at the ready. Insulin can easily go from refrigerator to tote in the morning. Don't forget a water bottle. A fun water bottle will remind you to hydrate throughout the day. **Prepack backpacks, purses, tote bags, gym bags, and briefcases and place them in your home's "launching pad."** A launching pad is one place in your home to corral all the items each family member must have before he or she leaves the house. An example of a launching pad could be next to your front door, at the entrance to your garage, or the house entrance or exit most used. **"Clean Sweep" your home.** Tidy kitchen. Empty garbage cans. Run the dishwasher at night and unload in the morning (if time permits). Toss in laundry or fold and put away clean clothes. These tasks are time robbers during the morning rush, so try to set aside time the night before to complete household tasks. **Shower the night before.** Have young children take a bath or shower in the evening, too. This cuts down on morning preparation time significantly. Extra bonus? A soothing bath will help you calm down and unwind after the day. If showering in the morning is a "must-do" and wakes you up, limit your shower time to 10 minutes. **Create your roadmap for tomorrow.** Go over your appointments and to-dos for the next day. A little bit of night time preparation will pay off big time in the morning.

Get to Sleep!

Do you get eight hours of restful sleep every night? A good night's sleep is one of the keys to good health. If you don't get enough sleep, you simply may not feel your best. Recent research has shown that lack of sleep can contribute to pre-diabetes. Also, people confuse fatigue with hunger and tend to eat more (and even binge eat) when they are sleep deprived. This can lead to weight gain as well as an increase in blood sugar levels.

Do you wake up constantly during the night because you need to urinate? Frequent urination during the night might indicate that your blood sugars are high. Don't just assume you are urinating more because you might have started to drink additional fluids.

Do you snore during the night? Snoring may be an indication that you suffer from sleep apnea. Sleep apnea can lead to a dangerous situation if left untreated. If you do not sleep well for any reason, please discuss the situation with your doctor. Your doctor might suggest a sleep study to help figure out why you have difficulty getting a good night's sleep.

If you have trouble falling asleep or you don't sleep through the night, check out our suggestions to help you get more shut-eye each and every night.

Tips and Tricks to Get a Good Night's Sleep

Get on a Regular Routine

Go to sleep at the same time every night. This routine should be kept on weekdays and weekends, especially when you first attempt to adapt to a specific bedtime.

Don't Fall Asleep on the Couch after Dinner

Fight the urge to close your eyes after dinner. If you fall asleep right after dinner, you won't accomplish your evening tasks and probably won't sleep through the night. You also might forget to take your evening medication or skip blood sugar testing. Remember that your bed is your designated place to sleep. Your couch is a place to sit and watch TV, read, and socialize. Once you agree to sleep in your bed, you'll probably be less likely to fall asleep before bedtime on the sofa.

Wake Up at the Same Time Everyday

Want to keep a good sleep rhythm? Wake up at about the same time every day. If you change the time you wake up or go to sleep too often, your sleep schedule will suffer.

Avoid Caffeine and Alcohol

Limit your consumption of coffee, tea, and other caffeinated drinks such as colas. Remember, even many diet sodas have caffeine. Try not to have any caffeine after the late morning hours. Substitute water with lemon, lime, or cucumber for caffeine-containing beverages. Also, limit the amount of alcohol you drink. It will disrupt your sleep cycle and could cause dehydration.

Beds Are for Sleep and Sex

It might sound funny, but if you only use your bed to sleep and make love, then the bed will have a specific purpose. Of course, you could also read a good book (or a boring book) in bed before turning out the lights. Keep your bed off limits for work, eating, or any other tasks.

Keep an Evening Routine

Plan out an evening routine and stay with it. Of course, certain evenings might require car-pooling with children, late nights in the office, or dinner out with friends. However, make sure that you stick to your routine once you're back at home.

Turn Off All Technology an Hour Before Bed

Turn off your TV, iPad, computer, or other technology an hour before you are ready for bed. Studies have shown that the artificial light sources in these devices actually trick our brain into thinking it's earlier in the day than it is. Turn your cell phone on vibrate and put it on your nightstand. Or, better yet, leave your cell phone in the livingroom and don't tempt yourself to check e-mails on your phone. You will reduce your stress and hopefully get a restful night's sleep.

Keep the Room Dark

Make sure that the shades are drawn and the lights are off. Cover lights on the cable box or computer if necessary. If any remaining lights bother you, try wearing an eye mask. Keep a flashlight on your nightstand (or next to your bed) so you can test your blood sugar if necessary during the night or check your CGM. If you are a parent of a child with diabetes, keep a flashlight next to your alarm clock so you can see clearly when you wake up to check his or her blood sugar during the night.

Try Lavender

Lavender has a very calming effect. Keep a lavender reed diffuser in your bedroom or throw some lavender bath beads into your evening bath. The calming effect of lavender can be very powerful.

Eat According to Your Preplanned Menu

You did a great job planning your meals for the week. Follow your menu to the best of your abilities. This process will help you avoid overeating unhealthy foods or consuming large portions in the evening that may prevent you from getting a good night's sleep. If one of your goals is to make healthier food choices, you'll feel accomplished (and not over-stuffed) when it's time to retire for the evening. Don't attempt to sleep with an overstuffed belly.

Keep the Noise Out

Have you ever tried to fall asleep only to be startled by a barking dog or the roar of thunder? If noises regularly bother you, try wearing ear plugs. Ear plugs are easy to use and very comfortable. You can purchase inexpensive ear plugs in any local drug store. Another possibility, try a soothing white-noise machine to help muffle outside noise. White-noise machines produce a calming sound that may help lull you to sleep.

My Morning and Evening Challenges

Spend some time considering both your morning and evening routines. What morning chores could be made easier with some evening preparation? What evening tasks seem out of control? Are there things that regularly keep you from getting a good night's sleep and leave you feeling less than energetic the next morning? Take a few minutes to jot down problem areas in your personal routine and, using the information from this chapter, brainstorm some solutions. It's no secret, better organization means less stress both in the morning and evening!

Problem Area 1 _____
Possible Solution _____
_____
_____

Problem Area 2 _____
Possible Solution _____
_____
_____

Problem Area 3 _____
Possible Solution _____
_____
_____

Problem Area 4 _____
Possible Solution _____
_____
_____

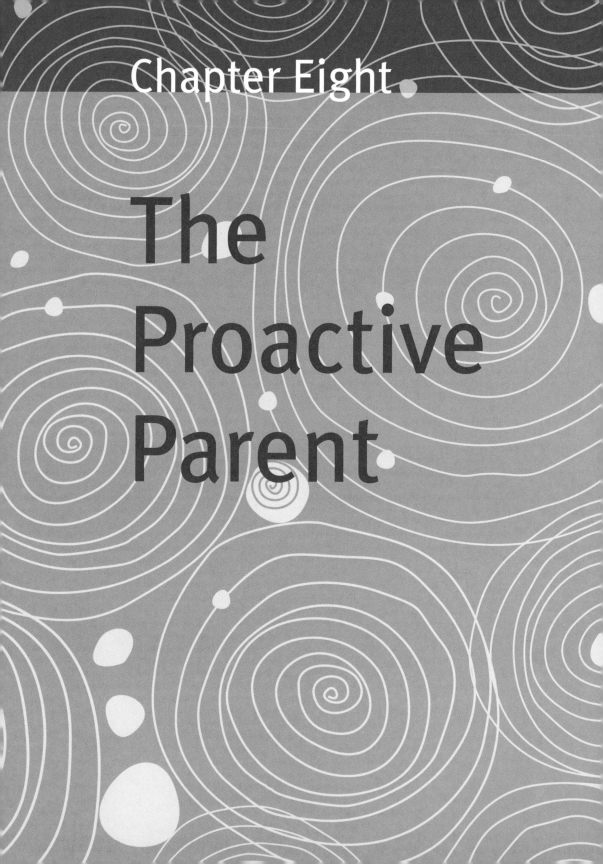

Chapter Eight

The
Proactive
Parent

AS A PARENT OF A CHILD WITH TYPE 1 DIABETES, you probably have many concerns. Do you worry about whether your child will be safe and well-taken-care-of when he or she is not at home and under your watchful eye? It's natural to be concerned about your child with type 1 diabetes when they are in school or at a friend's house. Finding the balance between being vigilant with your child's care and allowing your child to lead an independent life is forefront in every parent's mind. We can't tell you not to worry. All loving parents do. However, being proactive and arming yourself with the proper information, tools, and resources—for you AND your child—may give you a little more peace of mind.

Apps for Children

Topic	iPhone	Android
Med Reminders	Reminders, Pillboxie, MediSafe	MedCoach, MedMinder, MediSafe Virtual Pillbox
Carb Counting	Counting Carbs with Lenny, Eat Smart with Hope Warshaw	Counting Carbs with Lenny
PHR	Blue Loop	Blue Loop
Communication	Skype, FaceTime, Google+	Skype, Google+

Source: Adapted from *An App A Day* and *An App A Day for Health Professionals*, © 2012, Frederico Arts LLC; www.AppyLiving.com.

Managing Diabetes at School

Take a deep breath. With a proper plan, you can help ensure that your child's diabetes is well managed at school. It's certainly likely that your child's school has enrolled other children with diabetes over the years and therefore is not unfamiliar with what needs to be done. There might even be a teacher at the school who has type 1 diabetes or a staff member whose own child has diabetes. However, since every child and situation are unique, here are a few key steps to how to make your child's transition from home to school as seamless as possible.

Schedule a School Meeting

It is critical to ensure that the school and its personnel are comfortable and well educated about what will be expected of them. To do this, you should plan to meet with the school well before the school year begins.

Invite the school nurse, your child's teachers, school psychologist, school principal, *and* the physical education teacher to the meeting. Your goal is to discuss your child's DMMP, agree on the 504 plan, and review the care plan to be followed during the school day. This care plan will include regular daily maintenance in the classroom, physical education class, and recess, as well as how to handle emergencies, fire drills, lock downs, etc. Make sure that you provide information about your child's insulin and medication regime. Take the mystery out of blood sugar testing by showing the participants at the meeting your

Keeping Your Child Happy and Healthy at School

A diabetes medical management plan (DMMP), developed by your child's healthcare team, provides essential information on how school personnel should care for your child. It will also detail what your child can do independently and what he requires help with from a trained adult. For a sample DMMP, visit www.diabetes.org.

Used in schools receiving federal funding, a 504 plan spells out the accommodations that are necessary to ensure your child's needs are met and that he or she can succeed in the classroom. It will detail how the school's or teacher's policies are to be adapted to meet the needs of your child. Your child does not need to be having academic difficulty in order to be protected under Section 504. And remember, the school must also accommodate your child's needs during activities outside the classroom, such as sports teams or extracurricular clubs. Sample plans for children with diabetes can be found on the American Diabetes Association site and many others.

Distinct from a 504 plan is an individualized education plan (IEP), which is mandated by the Individuals with Disabilities Education Act. An IEP is put in place when a child has an identified disability that impedes learning to the point that the child needs specialized instruction in order to close the gap between the child's own academic achievements and those of his/her age peers. Most children with diabetes may not require an IEP.

For further information on special education law and advocacy for students with disabilities, please visit www.wrightslaw.com. You may also wish to contact a special needs consultant to determine whether a 504 plan or IEP is right for your child.

child's blood testing supplies, monitor, pump supplies, etc.

Don't forget the extracurricular activities. For example, if your child spends several afternoons rehearsing for the school theater production, attending chess club, or playing on an athletic team, make sure to include those teachers or coaches in the meeting. The teacher or coach in charge should be acutely aware of your child's diabetes needs and care.

Some schools share a nurse with other schools in the district rather than having one available all the time. Be sure to ask how the staff will meet your child's needs in the classroom and during activities such as field trips. Also, inquire as to the availability of a nurse if your child is staying after school to participate in activities. Inquire about how the school will communicate with substitute teachers. All substitute personnel should be made aware of the 504 plan for your child.

Prepare What to Bring to the Meeting

Here are some items to bring to the school meeting:
- Copies of pertinent medical notes, instructions (for example, how to treat a low blood sugar), reports, etc. that were given to you by your child's doctor or certified diabetes educator. These documents will provide the school team with a written guide to follow with all the instructions and contact information in one place.
- Detailed instructions for all diabetes supplies (including testing supplies, fast-acting source of glucose, extra batteries, and pump

or injection supplies, etc.) that your child will have or need at school are essential. School team members should be instructed on all aspects of your child's diabetes care as well as how to recognize and treat a hypoglycemic reaction.

- A signed consent from you allowing your doctors to communicate with the school. A Health Insurance Portability and Accountability Act (HIPPA) agreement signed by you or your child's guardian is also required. HIPPA was established to protect your or your child's medical records and personal health information. These forms are essential because, if a problem arises, the school staff may need to get information about your child's health quickly. Before the meeting you should determine the best method of communication between the school and your child's healthcare team.

Remind the School Personnel of Signs of Hypoglycemia (Low Blood Sugar)

- Trembling
- Fatigue
- Slurred speech
- Hunger
- Blurred vision
- Cold or clammy skin/pale face
- Dizziness/light-headedness

- Unexplained anger
- Tingling around the mouth
- Sweating
- Impaired cognition
- Fainting/loss of consciousness/seizure

- Signed and completed health forms. Make sure they are filled out thoroughly *before* the meeting. Remember to stay up-to-date on vaccinations and all immunizations.
- The American Diabetes Association (ADA) recommends that, in addition to the management plan, you give the school a packet with general diabetes information, including how to recognize and treat hyperglycemia and hypoglycemia. In reality, we are more concerned about a low blood sugar than a high blood sugar, but it's important to understand how to treat both. Also include emergency contact information for you and your caregivers, your child's doctor, and other members of the diabetes healthcare team.

Your School Checklist

These items are important to your child's health and safety.
- Knowing when snack and lunch times are for your child. This includes knowing schedules for early dismissals, late arrivals, and half days. It is critical to know when the usual schedule is disrupted so that you can plan ahead.
- Make sure your child wears his or her medical identification (ID) at all times. Although this is your child's responsibility, ask the staff if they could please check occasionally to make sure it wasn't removed. Chances are if you explain the importance of the medical ID, most teachers will be more than happy to check without making it too obvious. Remember to always thank your child's teacher for his or her assistance in this situation.

> We spoke to Jeff Hitchcock, the creator and editor of Children with Diabetes (CWD) (www.childrenwithdiabetes.com). CWD offers support to families dealing with type 1 diabetes. Jeff says, *"You'll find tips on how to talk to your child's classmates and their parents about diabetes as well as tips on communicating with school personnel. CWD actively engages people with diabetes (PWD), parents, grandparents, guardians, and siblings in the diabetes dialogue. If you need support or want to offer support to other families who have children with type 1 diabetes, please visit the CWD website."*

- Prepare an emergency kit for the nurse as well as any other classroom or activity your student will be at for great periods of time. Best to have in place by the first day of school. The list below will give you some key items for your kit.

Diabetes Beyond Your Front Door

Have you ever felt nervous as your youngster leaves the house in the morning? Whether they are going off to school, day camp, or even a play-date, chances are that you might be a bit uneasy about his or her diabetes management on the outside. The best way to prepare your child is to include them in the planning process. It's important to have your child communicate to you what they are comfortable taking

Diabetes Supply School Checklist

☐ Blood glucose meter, testing strips, lancets, and extra batteries for the meter

☐ Extra food, juice boxes, etc. (to be kept in the classroom, special classes such as art, physical education, and the nurse's office)

☐ Insulin, syringes/pens or extra pump supplies, including extra batteries

☐ Wipes

☐ Glucose tablets or other fast-acting source of carbohydrate

☐ Glucagon emergency kit

Note: Food and fast-acting sources of carbohydrate should also be kept in other areas where your child might receive services such as speech therapy.

Check throughout the year to make sure that none of the items have expired and then remove the supplies at the end of the year, restocking in the fall.

responsibility for and what they need assistance with. Being prepared will allow you and your child to be calm and confident all day long.

- Your child should have his own portable diabetes toolkit. It should include any essential on-the-go supplies that they need, such as meters, test strips, insulin, wipes, and fast-acting carbohydrates (glucose tablets or the like). Label the inside of the kit with your child's name and emergency contact numbers. Adhere a label to the toolkit with a list of everything that goes inside so that the kits are always stocked and ready to go.

- Make sure your child knows who their go-to person is— the person who is in charge of their care if they need help when they are away from home.

> Create a second toolkit as a backup in case the main kit gets left behind or lost.

- Have all their supplies and snacks portioned and labeled with the accurate carb count. This will keep the guess work out of measuring if your child is not in a place where they can measure quickly or accurately.

- Make sure your phone number is preprogrammed in your child's cell phone. Don't rely on their memory. If they are scared or feeling unwell, they might not remember how to reach you. These phone numbers should be programmed under Mom or Dad. Add an additional in-case-of-emergency (ICE) number to grandparents or other caregivers for additional backup.

- For an older child, teach them to set alerts on their cell phones for reminders. If they prefer, a medicine alarm watch specifically designed for children is an alternate option. Teach your child how to set the watch as a reminder to test blood sugar. www.epill.com or www.watchminder.com are great options.

Preparing Your Child's Caregiver

You might feel nervous and very uneasy the first time you leave your child in the care of someone else, even if it is in your own home or for a short period of time. When you are ready, you will find a caregiver or family member you trust when you are separated for the first time. In order to build confidence, start out slowly. Try leaving your child for no more than an hour the first time. Stay close by. This will make the transition of separation much easier. Remember, you can go back if you need to!

> Is your young child a lover of all things electronic? Introduce him or her to the app Carb Counting with Lenny. Your child can browse photos of common foods to learn how many carbs are in each or play games for points guessing if certain foods have carbs.

- Schedule a phone conversation or face-to-face meeting with the designated caregiver a day or two prior to the event to go over all instructions. This should be done regardless of whether your child is being taken care of in your own home or at friend's or relative's. This will allow quiet time to make sure all instructions are understood and there is ample time to ask questions.
- Prepare an instruction sheet regarding testing procedures, blood glucose targets, and how to treat hypoglycemia. Include the contact names and numbers for your pediatrician, endocrinologist, certified diabetes educator, and pharmacy. Laminate the instruction sheet and post it on the inside of the cabinet door or directly on top of the supplies in a drawer. Make sure grandparents, caregivers, babysitters, and even siblings are familiar with it. If your child will be taken care of outside your home, e-mail the instruction sheet a few days ahead of time so the caregiver has plenty of time to review and ask questions.
- Consider using the app Blue Loop. Your caregiver can update your child's information—the most recent blood glucose reading or dinner time carb grams—and then you can view in real time. You can set customized text messages to remind your child to check their blood sugar and it lets you know when your child has taken action.
- Keep fast-acting carbohydrates (such as glucose tablets) at friends, relatives, and babysitters' houses. Keep it in a drawer or cabinet that's within your child's reach. This will put everyone at ease.

Does your child spend a lot of time at a friend's house or at the neighbor's? Prepare a one-page information sheet with testing procedures, blood glucose targets, and how to treat hypoglycemia. Include the contact names and numbers for your pediatrician, endocrinologist, certified diabetes educator, and pharmacy and e-mail it to everyone. Suggest they tape it inside a kitchen cabinet or in another place that's easy to find.

Happy (Sleepaway) Campers

Sleepaway camp can be a wonderful experience for children with diabetes. It can boost their independence and self-confidence tremendously. Your child can have tons of fun at sleepaway camp and make lifelong friends in the process. While many parents choose a diabetes camp to help transition their children to independent living, many others want to send their child with diabetes to a mainstream camp, whether it's because other siblings, cousins, or friends attend or due to other connections to the particular camp.

If you choose a mainstream camp, it is important to do your homework to pick the right one for your child. Of course, if your child attends a diabetes camp, they will most probably have these systems already in place. But always ask questions and stay informed! Here are a few questions to get you started on the right path if you are considering sending your child to a mainstream camp.

- Does the camp have other children or counselors with diabetes?
- Will camp counselors and staff know what to do in the event of an emergency? Will they welcome and embrace your child, even though he or she will need extra care?
- Is there a nurse or medical personnel available at the camp?
- Is any of the camp staff educated in diabetes management? Are they willing to learn?
- Will the camp allow your older child to give themselves their insulin (or bolus) as needed? Will an informed staff member agree to assist your child as needed?
- How will your child adjust his or her insulin during active periods?
- Who will help your child check his or her blood sugar at night?
- Does your child or a staff member at the camp know how to monitor diabetes testing supplies in the summer heat?
- Will there be appropriate snacks and beverages readily available for your child?
- Who will accompany your child when they go out of camp on overnights, outings, or excursions?
- Can glucose tablets and juice boxes be kept in the bunk (with easy access) for your child?
- Will your child always have access to his or her cell phone? Does the phone have service if the camp is in a rural area?

How to Prepare for Camp

- Don't just speak to the camp director, but ask to speak to the members of their health and activities staff. It's important to set up those lines of communication.
- Ask to speak to parents of other children with diabetes who have attended the camp. They are a wonderful resource and will hopefully put your mind at ease. Many camps may not give you this information directly. You can request that the family contact you.
- Ask if you (or your child's certified diabetes educator/registered dietitian-nutritionist) can look over the meal plans and menus before your child goes to camp. If there are better food choices for your child, you will be able to try to put those in place before camp begins. Discuss all dietary issues with the camp before the summer begins (such as lactose- or gluten-free choices). Be prepared to supply dietary guidelines, recipes, and nutritional suggestions to the camp and dining hall upon your initial discussion. Note: A children's diabetes camp may not discuss menu options with you as it is assumed that meals are properly planned for children with diabetes.
- Prior to the start of camp, set up a detailed blood sugar monitoring schedule with your child and the camp. This schedule should consider ALL daily activities, including sports and evening events. Remember to ask about any changes in schedule, especially those affecting mealtimes.
- Pack and send to camp DOUBLE the amount of supplies you think

your child will need. Always better to send more than less. Check in with the medical staff prior to visiting day so you have plenty of time to gather supplies to bring.

- Since many camps include water activities, packing supplies in waterproof bags will help protect them.

With proper organization and preparation, your child may have a wonderful summer. Of course, camp can be a difficult transition, especially if your child has diabetes. If you decide that sleepaway camp is the way to go, visit mainstream camps as well as diabetes camps. You'll have the information you need to make a final decision on where your child might spend the summer.

Off to College with Diabetes

Do you have a child with diabetes who is approaching college age? Leaving for college is such an exciting time for young adults and their families. However, it's an especially scary time for you if your child has diabetes. For some, it is the first time he or she is away from mom and dad and needs to learn to truly manage his or her diabetes. This is a huge transition, but with detailed preplanning and organization, your child can learn to be more independent and manage his or her diabetes.

Getting Started

- When you and your child visit colleges, make sure to stop at the health centers as well. If possible, make an appointment to meet with the doctors, nurses, or health center staff to discuss your child's diabetes care.

- Ask your child's doctors (and healthcare team) for recommendations for doctors in the town or nearby city where your teenager is attending college. Make sure to leave plenty of time to transfer records and make appointments before the start of school.
- Find the closest pharmacies, including one that is open 24 hours a day. Arrange to have your child's diabetes care prescriptions available to be filled there.
- Network! If your child will be attending college far away, find a friend of a friend or other adult who can act as your child's emergency contact.
- Make sure your student signs all the necessary paperwork that allows you to discuss their care with the health center and local doctors in case of emergency. Once your student turns 18, you are no longer legally allowed their health information unless they give permission for you to do so.
- Call your insurance company. Make sure you are familiar with their out-of-state coverage as well as how they cover emergency situations.
- Make multiple photocopies of insurance and prescription cards. Have your student keep the originals in their wallet and copies in their dorm room in case their wallet is lost or stolen. Parents should keep a set also.
- Discuss with your child how you will communicate with each other. Make it perfectly clear that you want to be kept in the loop

regarding his or her diabetes, especially during the first semester. Who will order supplies? Set up clear procedures ahead of time. Keep the lines of communication open, nonjudgmental, and clear.

Check out the College Diabetes Network (CDN) to find a chapter on your campus. Chapters are created and run by students with a focus on peer support. The organization supports the chapters and students by providing the most up-to-date information that relates to students' lives. For more information, visit collegediabetesnetwork.org.

College Campus Checklist for Your Child

Here are some of our favorite tips to share with your college-bound teen.

- Meet with your resident advisor immediately to go over emergency procedures and other protocols.
- Contact your roommate as soon as you receive his or her information. Tell them about your diabetes and explain the signs and symptoms of hypoglycemia. Make sure you are both comfortable with each other as roommates. Once you are sharing space, inform them where you keep your diabetes supplies, fast-acting sources of glucose, and emergency contact information.
- Rent or purchase a small refrigerator for your dorm room for

supplies and snacks. Clearly label all your food and snacks so that your friends and roommates know not to help themselves to your stash.

> For college kids, www. DrinkingWithDiabetes.com offers nonjudgmental information about the impact of alcohol on people with diabetes. This is a must-have resource.

- Store double the amount of supplies you think you will need. Stash supplies in every bag and coat you use so you are never without.
- Wear your medical ID at all times.
- Make sure your friends and classmates know you have diabetes *and* what to do in case of an emergency, especially if you are out together at a party or other social function.
- Have two blood glucose meters in case one malfunctions. Always keep extra batteries on hand as well.
- Keep a sick-day kit on hand stocked with plenty of glucose tablets, Gatorade, juice boxes, and extra diabetes supplies. Better to have peace of mind that you have all you need when not feeling well.

Going to College with Diabetes: A Self-Advocacy Guide for Students is a free online resource from the American Diabetes Association designed to ease the transition for college students with diabetes. The guide helps students learn to navigate everything from the admissions process to life with diabetes on campus, and everything in between. The guide is available online at www.diabetes.org/assets/pdfs/schools/ going-to-college-with-diabetes.pdf.

To close out our chapter on caring for children with diabetes, we are honored to include a few inspiring and heartfelt suggestions from fellow members of the diabetes type 1 community. These parents share your fears, hopes, and dreams. With improved organization and communication, they gained confidence and raised empowered children. We hope that you will identify with these stories of triumph and promise.

The Karlya Family

Tom Karlya (aka "diabetes dad" to the diabetes community, www.diabetesdad.org, www.dLife.com/diabetesdad), VP of the Diabetes Research Institute, says "*learn everything you can about diabetes.*" He and his wife Jill have two children with diabetes, a daughter Kaitlyn and son Rob, as well as a son TJ who does not have diabetes.

Tom shares, "*When Kaitlyn first when off to school, Jill made sure that everyone was on the same page with managing her diabetes. We also wanted to make sure that she was included in all of the activities at school and after school. No child should ever be left out of activities because of his or her diabetes. Playing soccer or hockey is one thing. Playing soccer or hockey with diabetes is something else entirely. Our kids do everything with diabetes. Don't try to convince your kids that you know what it's like to have type 1 diabetes. They know that you don't have it. Conversely, they don't know what it's like to be a concerned and responsible parent who has a child with type 1 diabetes. If a child tells you that it hurts to take a shot, don't tell them that it doesn't hurt to take the shot. Listen to him or her. Let the child know that they can do anything they want with diabetes. There are no limits. I hear some parents say 'I don't let my child* swim because they have diabetes.' I point to Olympian Gary Hall. He won more metals after his diagnosis of diabetes than before. I told Kaitlyn, and eventually Rob, that we would do all we could to find a cure for diabetes. Being active with the Diabetes Research Institute (www.diabetes research.org), we wanted them to never lose hope that so many are continually trying to end this disease once and for all."

Tom and Jill put together a beautiful letter to share with Kaitlyn's classmates and their families. This type of letter is a proactive way to stay organized and share some of your concerns. Be proactive! Try using this letter as a template for you and your child.

Dear Parents & Guardians of Mrs. _____'s Class,

I am writing to you today about our daughter, Kaitlyn, who will be a classmate of your child this year at _____ Elementary. Kaitlyn is just like your child in the way she plays, laughs, and sings. Unlike your child, however, Kaitlyn was diagnosed with type 1 diabetes just about this time four years ago.

The first and most important thing you need to know is that no one can "catch" diabetes. It is what is commonly called an auto-immune disease. The beta cells that are normally produced by the pancreas were attacked by Kaity's own body and insulin is not created anymore. It is a disease that is born in children and magnifies itself sometime in the life of the child. Kaity was 2 when she was diagnosed. It cannot be passed from one human to another in any way.

Kaity has accepted, in many ways, her lifestyle. The diet she has to follow, the 2–3 daily injections of insulin, and the 5 blood tests she has to do every day have all been integrated into everything else that a 6 year old does in their busy little schedules. Kaitlyn is just now starting to understand what may be waiting in her future and the complications this dreaded disease can cause. It is a little tough sometimes and that is partly why I am writing today.

It is crucial for any child not to feel "left out" of the many things that children do together. It is our hope that you might help us, with some minor adjustments, so Kaity is included in these special activities. For birthday or holiday parties, would you kindly include a plain cupcake with no icing? Some of the things she can eat in varying amounts are a cup of popcorn, pretzels, sugar-free (NutraSweet) caffeine-free soda, sugar-free gum, vanilla wafers, animal crackers, and other products that contain NutraSweet.

Last year some parents gave stickers, balloons, and coloring books in the "goody" bags at children's parties. Kaitlyn puts up with a lot and in most ways you would never know anything is wrong. When you meet her, you'll find that she is very much like every little girl with the same dreams and the same needs. With a little understanding, some adjustments can be made so she is not "left out" of any activity—that is the worst thing that can happen.

Thank you for your understanding and feel free to call me (at number) with anything you want to discuss. There really is no such thing as a silly question when it comes to dealing with diabetes.

Sincerely,
Jill and Tom Karlya

Annette and Ryan Maloney

Ryan Maloney was diagnosed with type 1 diabetes at the age of two. Now at the tender age of 14, he is a triathlete, distance runner, and stand-up paddle board competitor. Ryan is an empowered and confident young man who inspires other children (and adults) with diabetes. His parents are instrumental in helping him stay focused and organized.

Annette told us that even though Ryan was only two years old when he was diagnosed with diabetes, she worked on teaching him lifesaving communication skills. *"My husband and I knew it was important for Ryan to feel somewhat responsible for his diabetes even when he was a toddler,"* Annette said. *"Only close family members or friends watched him for even a short period of time when he was very young. We knew what went into organizing and monitoring this disease, and we didn't want to burden others. We learned everything we could possibly learn about diabetes and worked with Ryan so he could learn how to organize and manage his own disease. One of the hardest parts of having him take responsibility for his diabetes management is that we didn't want him to get burnt out at an early age. The first time he changed his infusion set was not at our request, it was completely on his own. I believe that he chose to do that on his own because we gave him the confidence all along the way to help manage his diabetes."*

"Ryan loved sports from a young age, and we've always encouraged him to be active and to keep control of his blood sugars. We make sure that coaches, parents, and teammates are aware of his diabetes. We know how complex the disease is and don't expect anyone else to fully understand the disease. But we do want coaches and teammates to recognize the signs of low blood sugar levels in case there is an issue when

we are not present at a game or a practice. He needs to be prepared and organized and uses a supply pack. You can never be 'over prepared' when you have a child with diabetes who is participating in extreme sports."

Phil and Joanna Southerland

When Phil Southerland was only seven months old, he latched onto his mother's breast and wouldn't let go. He wouldn't stop sucking. His mom Joanna had to constantly change his extremely urine-soaked diapers. Although Phil was Joanna's first child, she knew that something was very wrong. When Phil was diagnosed with type 1 diabetes, without a supportive partner, Joanna gave up her career. She rarely slept more than a few hours at a time. Joanna was a former fitness instructor and exercise buff who had started to numb the pain of dealing with a child who had type 1 with compulsive overeating. "*I started shoveling potato chips into my mouth,*" Joanna said. "*I became very overweight and depressed.*"

"*One day I just told myself to stop,*" Joanna said. "*Enough is enough. I want to be a role model for my child. It was a defining moment. I started to teach spin and exercise classes again. I would go to sleep earlier (right after putting Phil to bed) and wake up at 2 a.m. and again at 4 a.m. to test his blood sugar. I set up an organized routine of sleep and exercise. I began to feel a little better about myself.*

"*I went to a support group when Phil was a toddler. At one of the meetings I met a 27-year-old woman who already had retinopathy. She didn't follow her doctor's advice to organize her diabetes supplies and* did not routinely test her blood sugars. She ate what she wanted and did not properly organize her food shopping trips. I went home and started crying on my porch, 'Phil's going to be blind by the time he's five years old.'

"My dear neighbor heard my sobs, walked over to my porch, and promptly slapped my face! She told me to educate myself on the disease and do everything I could to empower my son and encourage him to take charge of his diabetes. Three weeks later I was in the supermarket and the same woman was in the checkout line with her mother buying a ton of candy and ice cream! Not a vegetable or source of protein on the conveyor belt. I began to think about how meal preparation and physical activity can help pave the way for Phil to manage his diabetes.

"Diabetes would not define my son's life. Phil never used his diabetes as a crutch. Phil has gone to a diabetes camp where the kids had never met a true jock before. Phil became a true inspiration."

The Oringer Family

Over the past twenty-five years, Robert Oringer has created, built, and sold a number of diabetes-related businesses. He got started with his first diabetes product, blood lancets, completely by happenstance, and when Robert started marketing blood lancets, he never imagined that his company, CanAm Care, would go on to blaze a trail in the U.S. retail pharmacy market as the first company to offer a full line of private label (store brand) diabetes products. CanAm's line expanded over the years beyond lancets to include various hypoglycemia treatment products under the Dex4 brand name and insulin delivery products, such as syringes and pen needles.

In a strange turn, seven years after having sold his first boxes of lancets, Robert's two young sons were both diagnosed with type 1 diabetes. His older son Cory was three years old at the time, and his younger son Justin was diagnosed one month later at the age of nine months old. It was at that point in time that Robert and his wife Marla realized, very clearly, that their lives were changed forever, and together they made a decision that they would focus on diabetes from a family, business, and philanthropic perspective.

Robert explains, *"As a business person, I always look for ways to solve problems, and with experience I've learned that the most powerful way to do so is by building and being part of a team. My wife and I realized very early on the importance of applying our efforts together as teammates. It didn't take long for us to realize that, with diabetes, a team of three, four, or more could get a lot more done than a team of two. Given that we had two boys with diabetes, we have always tried to figure out how to expand our team with others we could teach and trust."*

Robert shares tips on building your diabetes team:

- Organizing your "home diabetes team" is incredibly important. You can go from one person with two hands to two people with four hands. Add in a grandparent, reliable babysitter, or close and trusted friend, and you quickly have six hands or eight hands to help with your child's diabetes. Find manpower! Don't push grandparents or friends away—recruit them, teach them, equip them, thank them, and reward them. When your child is first diagnosed, you might feel like it's too much work to train a grandparent or trusted relative to test blood sugars or be on the lookout for a low blood sugar. Find people who are interested in your child's welfare. Not everyone will be, but many will.

- There are diabetes problem-solvers in schools and in diabetes camps. Speak to your child's teacher about your child's diabetes. Some teachers have had previous students with type 1 diabetes. There might be a teacher in another classroom who has a child or former student with diabetes. That teacher could be an important part of your team!

- Stay current with technology and use it wherever possible. Over the past ten years, smartphones have helped us dramatically improve our ability to communicate with our children about their diabetes—simple texting of blood sugar numbers back and forth while a child is out with friends can provide freedom to the child, balanced with security and confidence. And beyond the communication aspect, the broad technology of smartphones can be leveraged for providing reminders, data tracking, calculating, location-based services, and many other tasks useful for better diabetes management. Almost amazingly, recent video chat technology built into today's smartphones can allow parents to go beyond just communicating blood sugars, but also allow parents to "see their child," which allows for even better communication. As a child agrees to stay in close contact via a smartphone and report blood sugars, they will develop more confidence and feel more empowered.

Great advice, Robert!

Chapter Nine

Organizing Your Medical Paperwork

What the world really needs is more love and less paperwork.
PEARL BAILEY

AH, THE DREADED PAPERWORK. It just doesn't stop piling up on a daily basis, right? And now add to it the endless notes from doctors' visits, medication logs, lab reports, e-mail correspondence, and insurance claims—it feels like you need a life jacket just to keep yourself from drowning in it. Hang on! We're here to rescue you!

The key to staying on top of managing and maintaining your medical paperwork is to create easy and efficient systems that work for you. How do you know what works for you? Get started by asking yourself the following questions:

- Are you a piler or filer? Color-coder? _____
_____
_____

- Do you already have a system that works for you to organize and manage paperwork, such as bills and other household-business information? If the answer is yes, then why reinvent the wheel?
_____
_____
_____

- Will others in your household need to have access to this information or are you the sole keeper?
_____
_____
_____

- Do you want this information to be portable so you can quickly grab what you need for doctors' appointments? Will you be able to carry your important information between home and work?

  _____

  _____

  _____

- Do you have ample space on a desktop, in a file cabinet, or bookshelf to store binders, files, etc?

  _____

  _____

  _____

- Are you tech savvy? Do you prefer to store all your information electronically?

  _____

  _____

  _____

By asking these questions, systems will naturally form. Just remember that there is no right way to maintain and organize records and documents. Whether you use a paper system, electronic software, or a combination of both, choose a method that works best for *you* and your lifestyle! And the method that works best for you is one that you can comfortably set up, maintain, and access. Choose one that provides you with ready access to the information you will need when you need it and, most critically, doesn't stress you out.

Apps for Paperwork

Topic	iPhone	Android
Paper File	Evernote, Dropbox, Google Drive	Evernote, Dropbox, Google Drive
Camera	Camera	Camera
PHR, EHR	drchrono EHR, Kareo EHR, MyChart, Mayo Clinic Patient, Acumen EHR, EHR Stimulus Calculator, IQMax Mobile, Allscripts Remote	drchrono, onpatient Medical Record PHR, MyChart, IQMax Mobile, Allscripts Remote
Appointments	ZocDoc	ZocDoc
Calendar	Awesome Calendar, CalenMob	Google Calendar

Source: Adapted from *An App A Day* and *An App A Day for Health Professionals*, © 2012, Frederico Arts LLC; www.AppyLiving.com.

Sort through the Sea of Medical Information

Before you get started, it's important to understand that your medical papers should be grouped into two basic categories—*Reference* and *Current*. Reference documents are papers that you want to keep for future use or referral but no longer need to access regularly or use on a daily basis. Your current papers are documents that are active and that you refer to consistently and need to keep handy. This categorization will be essential for you when you set up your organizing systems. Let's take a look at what falls into each category.

Reference Documents
- Medical history
- Old insurance policies
- Old flex spending information (if applicable)
- Settled insurance claims
- Old lab reports
- Paid medical bills and explanation of benefits forms (EOBs)
- Notes and correspondence
- Old food and exercise journals
- Past blood glucose logbooks or blood glucose monitor/CGM data
- Printed materials from diabetes groups or conferences

A general rule of thumb to follow is to keep your current records for one year in your active files, then move them to your less accessible reference files. A good reminder is to move your medical files to the reference files when you gather your tax documents for the year.

Current Documents
- Most recent insurance policy for medical, dental, and vision
- Current flex spending receipts (if applicable)
- Labs and test results
- Current blood sugar log or blood glucose monitor/CGM data
- Notes from doctors' appointments
- Medication log
- Recent food journal and exercise log

We asked Mary Ann Hodorowicz, RD, CDE, and Certified Endocrinology Coder, to share her expertise on medical paperwork. Mary Ann is a member of The American Association of Diabetes Educators (AADE) Board of Directors and an expert on medical reimbursement. Mary Ann says, *"It is easier than you think to organize your health plan documents (bills, statements, paid receipts, etc.) and medical documents from your providers. Keeping this paperwork organized and easily accessible is key to fully utilizing all your diabetes insurance benefits; insuring your bills are accurate and that your providers' charges are the lowest possible; insuring your payments are timely and affordable for your budget; maximizing your flex spending account at work, if available; and applying all eligible medical expense deductions on your tax returns."* Great and useful advice! Thanks, Mary Ann.

Filing It All Away

Keep your reference papers accessible, but they do not need to take up prime real estate on or in your desk. Store them in a file cabinet, on a bookshelf, or in portable file boxes or binders. Reference papers can be organized in many ways:

Categorically When filing medical records categorically, use hanging folders with large, clear tabs. This makes it easy to identify the file's contents and to retrieve the information you

167

need quickly. You can create file folders for each doctor or by types of records—EOBs, lab results, etc. Again, whichever works best for you.

Chronologically Set up your filing system by year. Once you have a chronological system, you'll be able to create and review your medical history naturally. So place all old claims, logs, and reports for each year in a separate labeled folder.

Color-coding Some people recognize color much faster than they can read text, so assigning colors to your categories can be an extremely efficient filing technique.

Binders Don't have ample file space? Prefer to have your records in view? Then create binders for your reference materials. Binders can be set up either categorically or chronologically as well. Store on a bookshelf for easy reference.

Going Paperless If you are tech savvy, there are many software programs and mobile applications to help you detail your medical information and records. If you are familiar with Google Docs or another cloud-based document format, this is a great alternative to a hard-copy record system. Or, consider scanning all your documents and then saving them to your computer. Create folders on your computer the same way you would for your file cabinet or binders.

Jakoter Health Tag (www.jakoterhealthorganizer.com) is a digital health history organizer. Their portable USB key chain offers an easy way to carry your personal medical information with you at all times or store past information with ease. Fill in your medical history on their predesigned templates. Jakoter Health Tag contains forms for just about everything that applies to your health history. You'll find forms that address your insurance information and immunizations, as well as everything in-between. When you go to the doctor, you can easily plug into their computer and share all your records.
Great for traveling, too!

Preparing for Doctor's Visits

You have scheduled your visit to your doctor. Good for you! You want to make sure to get all of your questions answered. We asked Mary Ann Hodorowicz for her thoughts on how you can get the most out of your doctor's visit. Mary Ann says, *"To get the very most out of each healthcare visit, bring a written list of all of your questions and concerns about:*

- *Diabetes care and treatment plan*
- *Insurance and provider bills and statements*
- *Lab reports and test results*
- *Any personal, financial, or family issues that may be impacting the quality of your life*

Never be embarrassed about discussing any of the above with any member of your healthcare team. They have your best interest at heart ... always. And know that they are the custodians of your personal health information, keeping it under lock and key."

Mary Ann also recommends that you take advantage of every medical/insurance benefit to which you are entitled. The two she recommends are the diabetes self-management education (DSME) program and also a diabetes medical nutrition therapy (MNT) program.

- A DSME program teaches you how to manage the ABCs of diabetes—A1c (a blood test that provides an average measurement of your blood glucose over a specific time period, usually three months), blood pressure, and cholesterol. Diabetes educators help you obtain the knowledge, skill, and confidence necessary for managing the key areas of diabetes self-care: healthy eating, staying active, coping, problem solving, self-monitoring, taking medications, and reducing risks. The last, reducing risks, includes preventing and slowing down the complications of diabetes, especially those involving the heart, veins, arteries, and nerves.

- Medical nutrition therapy is an essential intervention for all PWDs. During the MNT visits, a registered dietitian (RD) will counsel you on nutrition-related behavioral and lifestyle changes required to positively influence your long-term eating habits and health. Proven, evidence-based nutrition practice guidelines are used.

  In MNT visits, the RD:

- Performs a comprehensive nutrition assessment and determines your nutrition diagnosis.
- Designs an individualized meal plan that incorporates your food likes and dislikes, physical activity and exercise habits, eating schedule, types of diabetes medications you take, and even your cultural and religious dietary habits.
- Monitors and evaluates your progress toward meeting your blood glucose, blood pressure, blood lipid, and other metabolic goals (including weight, if needed).

"Taking charge of the 'business of diabetes' ... all these practical tasks ... in an organized manner will give you more of a sense of control and power over your diabetes. You will begin to feel proud—even amazed—that you've become the chief executive officer (CEO) and chief financial officer (CFO) of your diabetes affairs. And when you begin to reap the benefits of tapping into all your insurance benefits, you'll be even more delighted!"

Spot on advice, Mary Ann!

You can benefit from regular doctor visits, as well as participate in DSME and MNT programs. You'll be in charge of your diabetes organization sooner than you think!

Current Paperwork

Now that you have your old papers, documents, and forms filed and stored out of the way, it is time to focus on creating a system that allows you to have all the essential information you need at your fingertips.

Binders Are Your Best Friends

We admit it. We're binder girls. Leslie, in particular, stores **EVERYTHING** in binders. Her philosophy? It takes the remembering out of remembering. Meaning, if you are running to a doctor's appointment or to your child's school for a meeting, you don't need to think ahead as to what you may need. You can just grab the binder and go. What could be easier? Let's show you how!

Invest in a heavy-duty 4-inch binder, tabbed or pocket dividers, and sheet protectors to hold loose papers. You can customize the dividers based on your current information, but here are a few categories to get you started.

TAB 1: Copy of current insurance and prescription cards
List of medications with date, dosage, and frequency
List of all doctors on your team, lab, and pharmacy info
Copy of summary of insurance coverage
Drug and/or food allergies
Blood type

TAB 2: Logs including glucose monitoring, blood pressure, and weight

TAB 3: Recent medical history
    Immunizations
    Illnesses/surgeries/accidents
TAB 4: Lab and test results
TAB 5: Doctors' visits information
    Correspondence
TAB 6: Notes
TAB 7: Feel free to include a tab marked "School" if you want to keep your child's school forms or 504 in this binder as well.

Now that you have your binder ready:

- Include blank paper or a notepad in the binder so you are never caught without.
- Place a three-hole punched plastic binder envelope in your binder to corral prescriptions that need to be filled and pending lab orders. You'll find them in a hurry if they are front and center!
- Include a monthly calendar to jot down information such as when a symptom occurred or when you began a new exercise program.
- A three-hole punched pencil case comes in handy to hold Post-its, pens, paper clips, etc.

Keep any and all medical information such as meds, doctor info, allergy lists, etc. on a USB drive. Attach it to your key ring and mark it "medical info." Most emergency staff or doctor's offices will usually give you access to a computer.

- If you prefer to file your papers instead of placing them in binders, these categories can easily be transferred to hanging file folders.

Toting It Around

There are many other ways to keep your papers portable if you prefer not to use binders. Accordion files, plastic sleeves, or even a two-pocket folder will do. The choice is yours. But if you are looking for a few suggestions, here are our favorites.

Smead's MO File System. (www.smead.com) The MO file case goes from desktop to file cabinet to on the go. The case easily fits into a letter-sized drawer for storage, but the hand grips on either side make transport a breeze. Extra bonus? The file tabs are super-sized, making locating a file a snap.

Duo's 7-Pocket Accordion File Binder (www.amazon.com) Is it a binder? An accordion folder? It's both! This multitasking organizing tool combines a 3-ring binder *and* a 7-pocket accordion file folder for optimum organization. Extra bonus? It comes in an array of fun colors and elastic bands hold the file closed for extra security. No worrying about papers falling out.

Jamie Raquel's LifeStyle File Tote (www.officecandy.com) For all our fashionable friends, we have you covered. Combining the function of a file box with the stylish look of a handbag, you can tote your files in true style. The file rods inside hold letter-sized files and the large-sized open top provides easy view and access to all your files. This elegant tote comes in a plethora of colors from which to choose.

Staying on Top of Your Medical Bills

Have you tried to manage all your medical bills, account statements, EOBs, and diabetes all at the same time? You might feel challenged and overwhelmed at first. How do you stay on top of it all? Let's work together to create an easy and efficient system that will have you sailing right through the sea of medical bills. Try to read over the list a few times. Try one suggestion at a time. Soon you'll be on your way to a system that works for you.

- Set up a desktop filing system. You can use a vertical file holder, desktop file box, or even a magazine holder. Pick the tool that is right for you and your space. If you are short on desk or counter space, think "air space." Hang a vertical file on your wall, either in your office, kitchen, or even hallway. Need this system portable? Use a file tote, accordion file, or file folders.
- Create folders designated as follows:
  - Blank Insurance Claim Forms
  - To Be Submitted
  - Pending
  - Completed
  - To Pay
- As medical bills come in, place in the folder marked "To Be Submitted." Make copies of all medical bills before you submit them to the insurance company. This will help you track down claims or follow up on errors. (This folder and step may not be needed if your physicians submit claims directly to the insurance companies for you.)

- Once you submit the medical bill to the insurance company, place it in the folder marked "Pending." Make sure to write the date you submitted the bill on your copy.
- As the EOBs for a medical service come in, match them to the items in your "Pending" folder. This will give you a reference as to any billing errors, what services were provided, indication of what has been paid, and even create a health history.
- As you match the items up:
  - Place completed claims (that is, those for which nothing remains to pay) in the "Completed" folder.
  - Place items for which you have to pay any additional monies that the insurance company might not have covered (deductibles, etc.) in the "To Pay" folder.
- Review your "To Pay" folder on a regular basis (say, when you pay your bills). Again, make a note of any payments right on the copy.
  - Place the paid items in the "Completed" folder.
- Keep your completed medical EOBs in the "Completed" file for one calendar year unless you are in dispute over a specific claim.

Make sure to create a home for reminders and to-dos. For example, if you need to fill a prescription on Monday, follow up with the doctor on Wednesday, or call the insurance company next Tuesday, have one location for reminders. Anything that is pending or needs following up can be placed in your phone, written in your electronic or paper calendar, or jotted down on the wall calendar in the kitchen. It doesn't matter where you place it as long as you're going to see it every day!

Remember, to keep your paperwork from getting too out of control, commit to spending about 10 minutes once a week to go through, file away, put in binders, make calls, and complete any action you need to take. By doing so, you won't be overwhelmed. In fact, you'll gain peace of mind and you'll stay on course.

Notes _____

_____
_____
_____
_____
_____
_____
_____
_____
_____
_____
_____
_____
_____
_____
_____
_____
_____
_____
_____

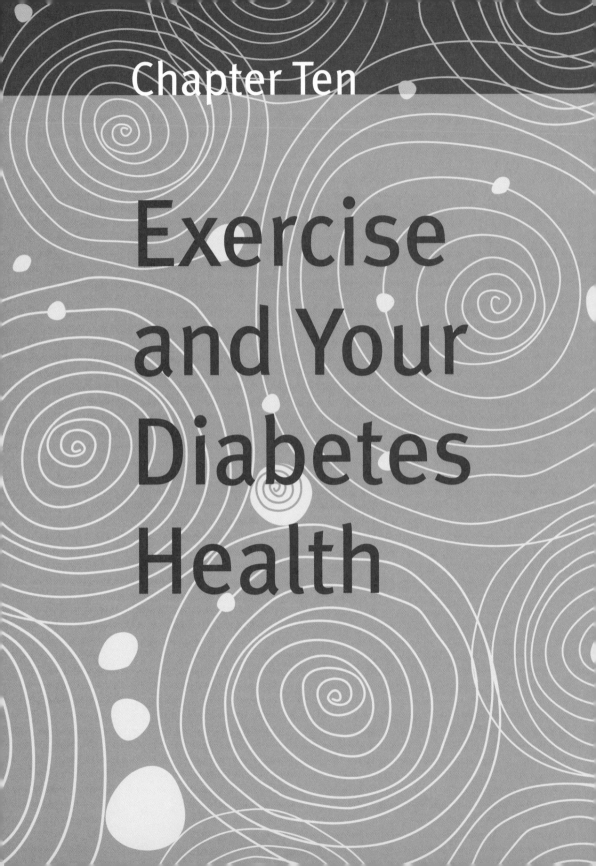

Chapter Ten

Exercise and Your Diabetes Health

Let's Move!

HAVE YOU EVER THOUGHT about the positive impact that regular exercise can make in your life? Your doctor or diabetes educator might have discussed with you some of the terrific perks at one of your visits. Perhaps you've heard that physical activity can help you control your blood sugar levels, reduce your stress, and lower your risk of heart disease. Have you also heard that exercise can help you control your weight and even help prevent nerve damage? Your doctor might have mentioned that regular exercise may reduce or, in some cases, eliminate the need for medications for some individuals with type 2 diabetes. It's all true.

But with so much to do during the day and evening, how do you fit exercise into your daily routine? Have no fear! Even if you don't like to sweat and have never worked out before, we can help you get started. Don't worry—with a proper plan and a few simple strategies, you will start to move more in no time. You don't need to run for miles or exercise for hours on end to get

Regular moderate exercise may help you:
- Control your blood sugar levels
- Improve how your body uses insulin
- Control your body weight
- Control your blood pressure
- Raise your HDL (high density lipoprotein or "good" cholesterol)
- Lower your LDL (low density lipoprotein or "bad" cholesterol)
- Build stronger bones and muscles
- Improve your balance and coordination
- Improve your flexibility and endurance
- Boost your mental focus and concentration
- Sleep better

some great results. All that matters is that you start to move. Remember, even if you exercise for 20 minutes, that's 20 *more* minutes of exercise than if you sat on the couch watching TV. Start small and, before you know it, you'll move more and start to reap the benefits of physical activity. You can do it!

Dr. Matt Corcoran is a board certified endocrinologist and founder of Diabetes Training Camp (DTC). DTC is a place where a PWD can learn to walk a longer distance, run a few miles, train for an endurance or multisport event, or anything in-between. We asked Dr. Corcoran about the benefits of exercise and diabetes management. Dr. Corcoran says, *"You can't take a pill or medication that comes even close to the enormous benefits that you'll get from regular exercise. At the heart of the matter is cardiovascular health. Did you know that heart attacks and strokes are the most common cause of illness and death for people who have diabetes? Diabetes is a metabolic and vascular disorder. People with diabetes who have never had a heart attack have the same risk of having a heart attack as those without diabetes who have already experienced a heart attack.*

"The good news is that a very modest amount of exercise will substantially reduce your risk of heart disease if you have diabetes. Did you know that if you start to walk for just two hours a week, you can reduce your risk of heart disease by 30 percent? It's true! If you increase the duration of your walk to three to four hours per week you can reduce your risk of heart

disease by 50 percent. That's right—walking 30 to 45 minutes per day, most days of the week, can cut the risk of heart disease in half! And, it is never too late. In fact, it does not seem to matter what your age is, sex is, race is, weight is, or how long you have had diabetes." If you want to learn more about Diabetes Training Camp, please visit www.diabetestrainingcamp.com.

We asked well-known author and certified cognitive coach **Ginger Vieira** for a few exercise tips. Ginger is 27 years old and has lived with type 1 diabetes and celiac disease since 1999. Ginger has won numerous power lifting contests and is a fitness enthusiast, but she didn't start out at her current state of fitness. She knows what it's like to feel overwhelmed with a diagnosis of diabetes. Ginger wants you to know that you should start to exercise slowly and build up your stamina and endurance. When Ginger speaks, we listen!

Ginger says, "*Are you overwhelmed when you think about exercise? Images of the 'perfect diabetic exerciser' inevitably pop into your head. It can be daunting to think you have to exercise every day. You might not even be sure where to start. But, here's a little secret, you don't have to be the perfect diabetic exerciser. Not tomorrow. Not next week. Not ever! Instead, you can gradually and carefully add exercise, or activity, or simple movement to your day. Maybe it happens every day or maybe just every few days. In any case, it'll be a step forward from where you are today. And maybe, in a few weeks or a couple months, you'll increase that to 20 minutes a day, or three days a week. Just start to move. You'll be glad that you did.*"

Exercise Recommendations

The American Diabetes Association (ADA, www.diabetes.org) and The American College of Sports Medicine (ACSM, www.acsm.org) have joined forces and put together exercise recommendations for people with type 2 diabetes. For more detailed information, go to www.ncbi.nlm.nih.gov/pmc/articles/PMC2992225/.

What do the recommendations mean for you?
- If you have type 2 diabetes, try to do more aerobic exercise. Do you like to walk, swim, or ride a bike? These are all aerobic activities that can be fun and may help you feel better emotionally and physically. You might even sleep better when you exercise early in the day. The recommended 150 minutes per week may sound like a lot at first. You can meet that goal if you exercise for 30 minutes, five days each week. Or you can work out for 20 minutes, seven days each week. Just start by walking your dog a little more or taking a stroll after dinner with your neighbor or friend. As Ginger says, "No worries if you start to exercise slowly." Soon you'll get into the groove and continue to move!
- Research shows that you may also benefit from some basic resistance exercise. Check with your doctor if you have eye or blood pressure problems. In certain cases, weight training can make those issues worse. Research shows that if you lift too much weight or position yourself incorrectly, you may hurt yourself and cause additional stress to your body.

- Try some resistance exercise (such as weight training) two or three times per week. Consider resistance exercise every other day. If you've never done resistance training before, you may want to work with a certified personal trainer. We realize that this can be costly, but you might find that it's a good investment. You don't have to commit to working with a certified personal trainer long term, but it might help you learn how to properly work with weights as well as use your own body as resistance. Does the idea of working out in a gym make you uncomfortable? Many personal trainers will work out with you in the comfort of your own home.
- Try a new type of workout. Soon you'll find an exercise program that you'll enjoy. You'll have fun once you find a program that boosts your energy and keeps you motivated. Remember to move your arms and legs. You'll increase your heart rate and burn more calories!
- Both the ADA and ACSM suggest that you use a pedometer along with personal goal setting (see chapter 1) to keep track of your steps. That way you can plan to move more and more as time goes on. Much more about that later! You can achieve your goal of increased physical activity if you simply take one step at a time.

Try to work up to exercising at least every other day. You're more likely to reap the full benefits of exercise if you work out more often.

Exercise Challenges

Make a list of all the activities you enjoy doing that will get you
to move. You don't need to exercise in a gym. Go outdoors and
walk. If you own a dog, maybe instead of taking your pet out for a
"quick pee," you can set an amount of time to walk or determine
a set distance goal. Turn up the beat and Zumba. Or, center yourself with yoga. If disco is your thing, then crank up the music and
start to dance. If you truly enjoy the activity, you are more likely
to continue to do it. It is that simple.

Activity 1 _____
Reason It Works for You _____
How Often? _____
_____
_____

Activity 2 _____
Reason It Works for You _____
How Often? _____
_____
_____

Activity 3 _____
Reason It Works for You _____
How Often? _____
_____
_____

Activity 4 _____
Reason It Works for You _____
How Often? _____
_____
_____

Before You Get Started Exercising

Always check with your doctor before you start any exercise program. It's especially important to meet with your doctor if you've been inactive for a long time. Your doctor might suggest a stress test or an electrocardiogram (EKG) before you start an exercise program. You should also make an appointment with your podiatrist and eye doctor. If you have certain diabetic complications (such as eye, foot, kidney, or blood pressure problems), your doctor may limit certain types of physical activities. So, if you haven't been active in a while, please schedule an appointment with your doctor today.

Check your blood sugar regularly before, during, and after you exercise. Physical activity uses blood glucose and, therefore, will affect your blood sugar levels.

> Consult your doctor or healthcare professional for specifics regarding carbohydrate, protein, fat, calorie, and fluid replacement before, during, and after exercise. Your needs may change based on your level of fitness, as well as the duration and intensity of your workout. You'll be glad you did!

- If your blood sugar is under 70 mg/dL, you are in a hypoglycemic range and should not work out until you are able to get your blood sugar into your target range. If your blood sugar is lower than 100 mg/dL, eat 15 grams of carbohydrate and re-test your blood sugar in 15 minutes. This is commonly known as the "15-15 rule." Repeat the process until your blood sugar level is within target range (usually 100 to 180 mg/dL).

- If your blood sugar is 100 to 180 mg/dL, you can start your workout! Please note that ADA-ACSM guidelines suggest that you can exercise if your blood sugar level is between 100 and 200 mg/dL. However, higher numbers may put more stress on your body when you work out, but this may depend on your overall state of fitness. The most important thing to do is to test. Don't assume that you know what your blood sugar is before you work out. Remember, the only "bad" number is the one you don't know!

- If your blood sugar is 200 to 250mg/dL or higher, be careful. It might be dangerous to start to exercise. Test your urine for ketones. If you are producing ketones, you should correct the situation before you start to exercise.

- If your blood sugar is 300 mg/dL or higher, do not exercise. If your blood sugar remains elevated, please contact your doctor. You can't start to exercise safely until your blood sugar is in a safe target range.

Be careful, hypoglycemia may be even more of a concern if you are taking insulin or an oral medication such as a sulfonylurea or meglitinide. Discuss your insulin or medication dosage with your doctor. Your doctor might also suggest changes to your injection site, depending on the type of exercise you plan to do.

What Are Ketones?

Ketones are chemicals that are produced when there isn't enough insulin for the high amount of glucose in your body. Ketones might be produced if you have been sick, had a recent infection, ate a large amount of carbohydrates, or don't have enough insulin. High levels of ketones can lead to medical problems associated with diabetic ketoacidosis (DKA) and can lead to coma or death. You can test for ketones with a finger prick or dipstick for your urine. Discuss the importance of testing for ketones when your blood sugar is above 250 mg/dL with your doctor.

Also, make sure you stay hydrated. Plan to drink plenty of water before, during, and after you work out. You might not feel thirsty, but plan to drink water to replace sweat losses and keep hydrated. Remember, exercise can affect your blood sugars for up to 24 to 72 hours, so you might experience a lower blood sugar several hours after working out. Sometimes your blood sugar might actually go up. Believe it or not, your blood sugar can go up after you exercise due to an increased production of certain hormones. Remember to test your blood sugar for several hours after you exercise.

Ginger says, *"Check your blood sugars often! Use your glucose meter during your workouts. It's the most helpful thing you can do for yourself! To help prevent lows and highs, check your blood sugar every 15 to 30 minutes—at least for the first few times you try a new type of exercise. If you are going low, at least you can catch it before it goes so low that you have to stop working out altogether."*

Signs of Hypoglycemia (Low Blood Sugar)

- Trembling
- Fatigue
- Slurred speech
- Hunger
- Blurred vision
- Cold or clammy skin/ pale face
- Dizziness/light-headedness
- Unexplained anger
- Tingling around the mouth
- Sweating
- Impaired cognition
- Fainting/loss of consciousness/seizure

Signs of Hyperglycemia (High Blood Sugar)

- Excessive thirst
- Weight loss
- Extreme fatigue
- Frequent urination
- Dry mouth
- Sweet or fruity breath odor
- Mental confusion
- Blurry vision
- High levels of ketones in the urine
- Shortness of breath
- Loss of consciousness/coma

Tony Cervati is an ultra-endurance athlete who has had type 1 diabetes for more than 36 years. Tony became the first person with diabetes to attempt the self-supported 2,750 mile Tour Divide mountain bike race from Banff, Alberta, Canada, to Antelope Wells on the Mexico–New Mexico border. He has competed in that specific event twice thus far, carrying everything he needed for the journey on his bike, including insulin, pump supplies, camping gear, fast-acting carbohydrates, water purification, etc. Tony knows how important it is to manage blood sugars, especially while exercising.

Tony says, *"I always keep my fast-acting carbohydrates, blood glucose testing supplies, spare batteries, and OmniPods in the same place in my bag. I place them in their respective spots, in the same quantity and order, each and every time before a ride. This way, in case I need them, I can locate them quickly. It also helps me to rectify whatever is amiss, and I can get back on the bike sooner. Nothing is worse than experiencing a low blood sugar and having to hunt around for a juice box or glucose tablets."*

Tony also says, *"When I'm on the bike and train regularly in season, I use approximately 35 percent less insulin. So my best advice is to test! Test! Test! Do not set yourself up for failure because you didn' t test your blood sugar."*

Apps for Exercise

Topic	iPhone	Android
Trackers	MyFitnessPal, RunKeeper, LoseIt, Map My Run, Map My Ride, Map My Hike, Map My Walk	Calorie Counter-MyFitnessPal, Map My Run, Map My Ride, Map My Hike, Map My Walk
Pedometers	MyLil'Coach, Monumental, Fitbit	Fitbit
Heart Rate	Cardiograph-Heart Rate Meter	Instant Heart Rate, Instant Heart Rate Classic
Blood Sugar	ibgStar, Vree, Glucose Buddy	Glucose Buddy, OnTrack Diabetes, Diabetes App Glucose Tracker
Water Tracker	8 Glasses a Day, Water Logged	8 Water, Water Log, Daily Water
Goals	App reSolutions, MyLil'Coach Goal Getter	
Music	iTunes, Pandora, The Play List	Pandora
Activity	HipHop Instruction, Country Line Dancing, Tango Book, Yoga, Couch to 5K	Tango-curso, Argentine Tango Exposed, Learn Country Line Dancing, Daily Yoga, Simply Yoga, Yoga For All, Couch to 5K

Source: Adapted from *An App A Day* and *An App A Day for Health Professionals*, © 2012, Frederico Arts LLC; www.AppyLiving.com.

Fit Exercise into Your Schedule

We know it can be a challenge to make exercise a consistent part of your life. Do you feel strapped for time? Does the drive to and from the gym add precious minutes to your already tight schedule? What can you do to make sure you fit exercise time into your routine? Here are our tried and true tips for exercise success!

Determine which days of the week work best for you. If you just started an exercise regime, you may want to schedule your workouts for alternate days. You may also want to mix weekdays and weekends, especially if you have more time on the weekends.

Next, figure out what time of day would be best for exercise. Are you a morning person? Do you think a morning workout will set the tone for the day? Or, do you think that an evening workout will help you unwind? Perhaps a lunch-time workout is the kind of midday break you need. The only "right" time to exercise is the time that is right for you. If you pick times that truly work for you, then you are more likely to follow through with your exercise plan.

Start slow. If exercise is new for you, don't plan hour-long sessions five times a week. Try to walk or lift weights (with your doctor's permission) for just 10 minutes.

> Do you have trouble falling asleep at night? Try to exercise earlier in the day. You might fall asleep faster and stay asleep longer.

If you lift weights (and use proper form) every other day, you may eventually feel more toned. You can gradually build from there. Increase the duration of your workouts or their frequency. Remember, regular exercise is a process. Keep going! You are strong and about to become stronger.

Set goals. Regular exercise is a goal for many people with diabetes. In the goal chapter, Jim Turner told us that one of his goals is to exercise more often. Jim is a busy actor, comedian, and diabetes advocate who knows that the only way he will exercise is if he plans to do it. He WILL DO IT and so will you!

We asked well-known author and PWD Gary Scheiner, MS, CDE, how he fits in exercise with his busy schedule. Gary is the owner and clinical director of Integrated Diabetes Services LLC. Gary says, *"I try to get some form of exercise almost every day of the week. With a wife, four kids, and a practice to manage, there are plenty of challenges to maintaining consistent workouts. The key is flexibility and planning. At the beginning of the week, I take a look at my schedule and decide when I can fit in a workout each day—some are in the morning, some in the evening. When I travel (which I often do to deliver lectures), I use the hotel's workout room, go for a run, or bring along a jump rope to use in the room."* Gary told us that he tests his blood sugars even more often when he travels. Great idea Gary!

Treat exercise like an appointment.
Schedule your exercise like you would a haircut or manicure. Write it in your planner, jot it on your calendar, or load it on your phone. Physical activity is one appointment that shouldn't be postponed or taken off the calendar.

Mix it up! Create a routine where you do different exercises on different days. Do aerobic exercise on some days and weight training or resistance exercises on others. What a great way to keep your routine fresh and fun.

Create a playlist. Exercise to your favorite tunes to keep you on track and motivated. Download your favorite songs and turn up that beat!

Have the clothing and equipment you need on hand for the various activities you like to do. Create a drawer or shelf space for your workout clothes. Assign a designated area to keep any equipment you need. No more excuses!

> Make sure to always wear your medical ID when you exercise. Carry emergency contact information in your pocket at all times.

> Set an appointment reminder on your cell phone or computer to remind you to exercise. Have the reminder go off 15 minutes before you plan to work out. That will give you enough time to wind down whatever you are doing and help you transition to your exercise time.

Enlist the help of a friend. We all need encouragement to stick to a fitness program. It's easy to hit the snooze button when it is just you, but much harder to leave a friend at the track first thing in the morning. And, you would be surprised how much faster an hour of exercise goes by when you're with a friend or partner than if you're alone.

Keep an exercise log. Write down how much you exercise. Also record how you feel when you work out. For example, do you feel energized and focused? Do you feel achy? Test your blood sugar and listen to your body. You'll become more aware of how much better you feel emotionally and physically once you start to move more. You don't have to be an Olympian to feel like one!

Reward yourself. After successfully working out for a specific period of time (for example, each week), reward yourself! Try not to reward yourself with food. Schedule a massage or manicure-pedicure. Take in a movie or concert. You deserve a reward for sticking with your exercise plan.

Get Ready! Get Set! Start to Move!

You don't have to go to a gym to increase your physical activity. If you enjoy going to a gym or working out with a personal trainer, that's wonderful! But you can exercise in your home or outdoors, too! The most important thing is to find an exercise routine that fits your needs. Now let's start to move!

- If you watch TV in the evening, multitask. You don't need to sit on

Diabetes Training Camp's very own Carrie Cheadle shares some of her thoughts on how to focus on your exercise goals. Carrie says, *"Your desire to exercise has to be greater than your desire to not exercise. When you're juggling family, work, and diabetes, it can feel challenging and overwhelming at times to add exercise into the mix. In the beginning, it can help to create an external reward system to help with your motivation to work out. For the first month, it may be motivating to give yourself a reward for each week that you accomplish your exact exercise goals. Then you may switch up your rewards structure. Add a reward each time you try something new or you meet your monthly goals. Think of rewards that complement the healthy behaviors you want to implement. Treat yourself to new workout clothing, work with a personal trainer for two months, or sign up for a new class! You deserve great rewards for your efforts as well as the enormous health benefits that come along with working out. However, in order to sustain motivation over time, you need to be intrinsically motivated as well. Be sure to add in exercise that sounds like fun—something that you would want to do regardless of the fact that it means you are also working out.*

If you do fall off the exercise wagon, don't give up! And please don't beat yourself up. Think of this as a lifelong endeavor and don't worry if you skipped a week or missed a month. Each time you get back at it, you increase your chances of strengthening your commitment to yourself and your health." Carrie's advice is honest and rings true for so many people with diabetes. Thank you, Carrie.

the couch to watch your favorite TV show. You can march in place, ride a stationary bike, or walk on a treadmill. Use light hand weights to get in a boost of strength training.

- Visit your local library to try a workout DVD for free. Once you know what you like, you can purchase one to keep at home. There are great fitness DVDs available for all levels of fitness.
- There are all kinds of smartphone apps for tracking your exercise routine, watching your progress, and setting goals. These apps are designed for everyone from hardcore exercisers to those just getting started. Look around for ones that fit your needs and personality.
- Stay physically active throughout the day. Remember to wear your pedometer so you can see how much you walked. A planned workout is fantastic, but moving more during the day can help improve your blood sugars and control your body weight. Make a few extra trips to bring up clean laundry or take newspapers to the curb and come back for the recycling bag. Take the stairs instead of the elevator at work. Ready

> Put a "step" in front of your TV. While you watch TV, walk up and down the exercise step. To burn even more calories, add light hand weights. Every time you think about heading to the refrigerator for a snack, do another 10 steps instead!

to unload the car? Walk back and forth to unpack the trunk. Before you know it, you'll get in a "chores" workout and you'll be glad you did.

- Keep comfortable, properly fitting sneakers, tennis, or walking footwear at work and at home. Put on your sneakers and walk for a few minutes when you have some downtime.
- Have your workout clothes ready to go. Keep your workout gear in the trunk of your car in a tote bag. If you joined a gym near your office, keep your gear at work.
- Stand more, sit less. Walk in place while you chat on the phone. Pace while you wait for your table at a restaurant. You get the idea. Keep moving!
- Wear a pedometer or fitness tracker. The joint statement from the ADA and ACSM recommends using a pedometer to monitor the number of steps you take every day. That will help you set a goal to take more steps and increase your physical activity level. If you currently take 1,000 steps per day (which is approximately half a mile), shoot for 1,100 by next week. By the end of the week, you'll walk more, burn more calories, and gain more control over your blood sugar levels.
- Park farther away. Instead of circling the parking lot while you look for the nearest space to the store entrance, park your car a little farther away. Soon you'll start to walk more and more every day.
- Do something different. Not everyone enjoys using a treadmill or stationary bicycle. Figure out what you like to do and start to do it!

For example, do you like to dance? Join a Zumba class or sign up for dance lessons. Turn the music up at home and dance in the privacy of your living room, if you're so inclined.

- Do you like to walk but don't want to walk alone? Check out local walking groups in your neighborhood. If the time is inconvenient, round up a few friends, coworkers, or neighbors and find a time to walk together. If you sit for too long, you may increase your chance of developing medical problems, such as blood clots. Once you find an activity that you enjoy, you'll be more likely to continue to exercise.
- Work out from your chair. Do you sit for hours on end at the office or in front of a computer? Try to get up and walk for five minutes every half hour. Soon you might even notice an increase in your concentration.
- Walk more, drive less. Do you go to the corner store for a carton of milk? Don't take the car. Walk or take a bicycle ride. You'll use less gas and burn more calories!

Must-Haves for an Organized Gym Bag

You will be well on your way to exercise success with a stocked and organized gym bag. Here is a checklist to help make sure you have everything you need. You might not need everything on this list. Take what you need for a successful workout!

- Exercise clothes (including shirt, shorts, athletic socks, athletic supporter, sports bra, and sneakers)

- Change of clothes for the day (don't forget a fresh pair of undergarments)
- Towel
- Weight-lifting gloves and/or belt
- Music player and ear- or headphones
- Water bottle
- Towel and washcloth (if you prefer your own)
- Toiletries (including soap, toothbrush, toothpaste, deodorant, shampoo and conditioner (and other hair products), body lotion, cotton swabs, razor, and shaving cream)
- Flip-flops for the shower
- Baby wipes
- Shower cap
- Makeup
- Plastic bag for dirty clothes
- Hand sanitizer
- Sports watch/pedometer
- Yoga mat
- Glucose tablets or other fast-acting source of carbohydrates
- Meter and testing supplies (check expiration dates)
- Healthy, nonperishable snacks. Some to consider—unsalted almonds or walnuts with raisins, natural peanut butter on whole grain crackers, natural almond butter on a rice cake, or a high-fiber granola bar

We asked Tony Cervati what he keeps in his gym bag. *"I keep my workout clothes and a spare tee shirt and socks in my gym bag. I'm always prepared for spills. I also have a spare glucose meter and test strips, fast-acting carbohydrate (a 20 oz. regular soda), a towel, antibacterial hand lotion, an extra OmniPod, insulin vial and syringe, my TRX equipment, an iPod, and my sneakers. I prepack everything the night before so I don' t have to rush (or forget anything) as I head out the door."*

Tony also has a separate bike bag for race day. *"I carry a bike bag on my back while training and racing. I have an otter box (a waterproof container) with my spare PDM (the "brains" of the Omni Pod), another otter box containing 2 spare OmniPods, insulin vial, syringe, and spare test strips, two bags of M&Ms, a tube, a multi-tool, spare derailleur hanger and chain links, four zip ties, 100 oz. hydration sack, rain jacket, a spare jersey, four AA and two AAA batteries, and a tire lever. This selection allows me the opportunity to adjust the length of my rides on the fly, be prepared for a diabetes-related emergency or equipment failure, fix any repairs, and soldier on in changing weather conditions."* Wow Tony! You are truly organized and prepared for race day!

Tap into Your Inner Athlete

Diabetes doesn't have to slow you down. Organize your schedule and plan your workouts so you can achieve remarkable goals. Check out some of these incredible athletes—who happen to have diabetes.

Will Cross has climbed the highest peaks on all seven continents. He has also walked to both ends of the earth. That's correct; Will has walked to both the North and the South Poles. Will climbed 15 unexplored mountains in Greenland and has gone on expeditions in Patagonia and the Sahara Desert. The fact that he's accomplished athletic feats that very few human beings have even dreamed about while having type 1 diabetes for more than 30 years is beyond motivating. Imagine having to adjust your insulin and massively fluctuating blood sugars at altitudes such as Mt. Everest! Will dealt with the stress on the body of high altitudes as well as the psychological stress of living off the land during other extreme and dangerous expeditions.

Will says, *"An unspoken advantage of diabetes is that we are required to plan in areas that other people don't always have to think about. We have to plan things out. We have to stay organized. But we also can use diabetes to give us huge payoff of an incredibly productive life. Embrace your diabetes. Don't get buried by it."*

Saul Zuckman is a 73-year-old gentleman with type 2 diabetes. Saul was diagnosed with diabetes 23 years ago and realized that he needed to adopt some healthier lifestyle changes. Saul says, *"The best approach* to creating new habits is to identify the habit that you want to create or a bad habit that you want to break!" Saul soon realized that regular exercise was the habit that he wanted to create and inactivity was the habit he wanted to break. Saul says "After my father-in-law passed away from complications related to heart disease and diabetes, I inherited his old ten-speed bicycle. Although the bicycle had a great deal of sentimental value, it used very old technology and was limiting my abilities as a rider. Soon I bought four new bicycles! I became passionate about riding and became a mentor for a bicycle program that worked with teenagers.

"My passion and skills for cycling continued to grow over the years. At the age of 70, I was selected to be on an all-diabetic eight-person team that did the Race Across America event, which is a bicycle race from San Diego, California, to Annapolis, Maryland. There were the eight of us who raced and we had a 21-person support team. I guess it takes a village to get a team of persons with diabetes across the country safely. At any one time, 24 hours per day, half the team was on the road while the other half was on rest status. The race team shared a standard-sized RV with crew members. This meant the living and storage quarters were very limited. Since we slept on the go, no motel stops, we had to carry all of our supplies. The bicycles, shoes, and helmets were shipped ahead to the starting line. We were each limited to no more than 12 pounds of gear! I needed to fit 10 days' worth of medications and diabetes supplies into a pillowcase-sized soft bag. Anything over the weight limit was shipped back home. Our team leader carried a small parcel scale to enforce this team requirement. This forced each of us to think through our personal requirements, delete the 'nice to have' but not essential items. I made a list (of essential supplies) and weighed each item on the list. I only used the exact same amount of supplies for days prior to the trip. This helped me organize my supplies and taught me how to be frugal with what I truly needed for the ride. The process was: select, practice, then adjust.

"Blood sugar testing was of paramount importance during the event. Each racer was required to test his blood sugar just before and after each racing leg, and before and then two hours after eating. Frequent testing became a habit. If it appeared that one of the racers skipped a test, the others would certainly remind him. This was required and not optional. If any of us experienced hypoglycemic (low blood sugar) and hyperglycemic (high blood sugar), it was addressed immediately. We constantly reminded each other about the importance of good blood sugar control. After all, we all relied and depended on each other for support and encouragement."

Saul is proof positive that regular exercise has no age restrictions. Ride, Saul, ride!

Tony Cervati provided the last thought for our chapter on exercise. "Competing in ultra-endurance length mountain bike events is very similar to living life with diabetes. You must plan your route ahead and be prepared for everything that might happen while on the bike. Once you start, make sure you're knowledgeable and flexible enough to adjust to the unknowns. Trust me, the unknowns of diabetes and exercise will jump right out in front of you. Always be prepared for every possible *situation. Every day could bring a new and exciting challenge. I keep my supplies organized and my knowledge about diabetes management up to date. Find something you like to do and do it. Don't worry about what someone else does to stay physically active. Once you find an activity that you enjoy, the sky is the limit."*

Activity Log

Start each week off with a fresh sheet and see if you can get closer with each passing week to the goal of 150 minutes of weekly exercise.

	Date/Time	Duration (mins)	Activity	Notes (low blood sugar, pain, etc.)	Blood Glucose Before	Blood Glucose After
Sunday						
Monday						
Tuesday						
Wednesday						
Thursday						
Friday						
Saturday						

Visit www.sprypubdiabetes.com to download a printable pdf of this activity log.

Chapter Eleven

Your Diabetes Travel Guide

DO YOU EVER TRAVEL for business or pleasure? If you have diabetes, you probably realize how important it is to have everything you need ready to go before you board a bus, train, or plane. Would you arrive at the airport without a plane ticket? Do you expect to stay at a popular hotel without a reservation? Of course not! You wouldn't travel to a beach in Aruba dressed in a winter coat or ski in a bathing suit. And you should never travel without your diabetes tools and supplies. So, while diabetes never takes a holiday, you can! Enjoy your well-deserved vacation. Go on your business trip with confidence. But remember that your ability to organize yourself and your diabetes supplies is a non-negotiable part of travel. Regardless of the purpose or length of trip or your destination, organization begins before you take off!

> Dr. Francine Kaufman, former president of the American Diabetes Association, is the Chief Medical Officer and VP at Medtronic Diabetes. Dr. Kaufman, also a Distinguished Professor of Pediatrics Emerita at the Keck School of Medicine at USC, says, *"Talk to your doctor about where you are going and how long you plan to travel. Make sure you discuss all of your travel plans with your healthcare team, including any possible medication or insulin adjustments."* Dr. Kaufman strongly suggests that you meet with your doctor at least 4 to 6 weeks before your trip if you require immunizations.

Preparing for Your Trip

Time Zones

If you plan to fly across time zones, your doctor or certified diabetes educator can help you determine how to adjust your insulin pump, insulin, or medications. If you plan to travel east-bound, you might have to adjust your insulin and meals for a shorter day. If you travel west-bound, you may need to adjust your insulin and food for a longer day. Insulin adjustment will likely be necessary if you plan to travel over several time zones.

> Ask your doctor for a letter on office stationery explaining that you have diabetes and detailing the list of diabetes essentials that you need to carry with you. Hopefully, your letter should help insure a smooth time through security lines.

Prescriptions

Make sure to obtain written prescriptions from your doctor for additional medications, supplies, and insulin. If you travel within the United States, try to use a recognizable national chain pharmacy (such as CVS or Walgreens). Make sure your prescriptions are updated in the database. This will allow you to go to any nationally recognized pharmacy and get medication if needed. The American Diabetes Association (ADA) also recommends that you contact the International Diabetes Federation (www.idf.org) if you need additional prescriptions in foreign countries.

Do you need information from a pharmacy while you are away from home? You can use an app to access many pharmacies on your smartphone.

Test Your Blood Sugar
Make sure your blood sugars are in target range before you travel. Test more often at least a month before you plan to travel to help

Keep all of your essential medical documents together in a travel organizer. There are plenty of plastic envelopes or pockets from which to choose that can help you corral your travel documents. Our favorite? We like the Travel Organizer by Smead (www.smead.com). You can use the three clear plastic-tabbed sections. Now you can sort all of your important travel and medical documents and keep all the important information right at your fingertips. Plus the secure front pocket keeps extra prescriptions right at hand.

improve your diabetes management. You will be more likely to enjoy your trip if you are less concerned about possible blood sugar changes while you are away from home.

Emergencies

Contact your insurance company to ask for a list of available doctors, hospitals, or urgent care centers in the area you will be visiting. Review your health benefits and get a list of any useful contacts before you travel. Contact the International Association for Medical Assistance to Travelers (www.iamat.org) if you have a medical emergency.

Climate Change

Insulin doesn't have to be refrigerated and can stay at room temperature for a period of time. However, if you are traveling to a very hot or cold climate, be aware that insulin can lose its strength if kept at extreme temperatures. So, when in doubt, keep your insulin refrigerated.

Traveling Overseas

If you are traveling overseas, drink only bottled water. Remember to avoid ice cubes made with tap water, as well. Also, be careful of street food and local markets. If possible, try to become familiar with the nutritional and carbohydrate content of local cuisine before you travel.

Footwear

Wear comfortable shoes or sneakers and socks that fit properly. If you find it difficult to walk or have problems with your feet, visit your podiatrist a few weeks before you travel. If you need assistance when you walk or have an unsteady gait, consider using a taxi or car service when you travel.

> Do you take insulin? Consider taking a bottle of regular insulin along in case of a sick day emergency as well as a glucagon kit. This is especially true if you are considering adventurous travel.

Check Out the Transportation Security Administration (TSA) Regulations

The TSA offers a travel helpline for passengers with disabilities and medical conditions. Call TSA CARES 1-855-787-2227 or visit www.tsa.gov/traveler-information/travelers-disabilities-and-medical-conditions.

American Diabetes Association

Review their web page for guidelines for air travel. It includes TSA regulations for people with diabetes. www.diabetes.org/living-with-diabetes/know-your-rights/discrimination/public-accommodations/air-travel-and-diabetes/

Airport Security and Customs

Become familiar with the security screening process at the airport before you go. Do they require a note from your doctor? Also be knowledgeable about the customs and security procedures for your destination country. No need to be surprised when you get there. Always do your homework beforehand.

Travel Tips from the Experts

We thought we'd share some tips from some well-known frequent fliers.

Nat Strand, MD, is an Assistant Professor in Clinical Anesthesiology and a practicing physician of interventional pain management at Keck School of Medicine at USC. *"Organizing my diabetes supplies for the Amazing Race was the first, and probably most difficult, challenge of the entire adventure. When I found out I was going to participate in the Amazing Race, I was elated. The next thought I had was how am I going to pack for this? Those of you who watch the show are familiar with the fact that all we have is a backpack. This one backpack has to hold everything we need for an entire month. Clothes for deserts, gear for icy mountains, and everything in-between. Packing for a person without diabetes is always a challenge when traveling. Using only a backpack for all of my diabetes supplies in addition to proper clothing for the race seemed impossible. But when you have diabetes, you need to make it all work! And so I did.*

"The first thing I did was make a list of all of my daily diabetes

supplies. I needed my pump, reservoirs, infusion sets, alcohol swabs, insulin, syringes, batteries, glucometers, test strips, lancets, continuous glucose monitor (CGM), charger, glucose tablets, glucagon, and extra batteries. I tried to think about what I would need if I were hyperglycemic, what I would need if I were hypoglycemic, and what I would need if I was in target range. Next, I estimated how much I would need for four weeks. Then I doubled it. It's always better to have too many supplies. You never know when you are going to accidentally pull out an infusion set, run out of batteries, or drop your test strips down an elevator shaft. (Hey, it has happened!)

"When I was satisfied with the supplies I had on hand and the amount of them, I laid them all out on the floor. It was more than would fit into my backpack—and that is without any clothes! This is where organizing truly came into play. I took my pump supplies out of their bulky packaging and placed them in a zippered bag. This isn't sterile, of course, but it did save a lot of space. The next thing I did was pack more test trips into each test-strip bottle. I figured out that about 50 test strips fit into a 25-strip bottle. I put my glucose tablets in zippered bags as well. I like to use makeup bags to hold my stocks of supplies. Syringes, insulin, alcohol swabs (all of the injection supplies) go in one makeup bag. Testers, strips, lancets, all go in another bag. And then I have one 'daily bag.' A diabetes organizing system that has all of the supplies in one place, so I only have to go to one spot to get everything I need. There are several systems out there. I chose to use the Dia-Pak Deluxe Diabetic Supply Organizer, and it was perfect. I would refill it every night or two from my backup supplies and keep that packed at *the top of my backpack for easy access.*

"The best part about the Amazing Race is that I now know that with good planning anything is possible. That was the most organized I have EVER been with my diabetes. And it definitely made things not only doable, but easier in a lot of ways than things had been at home. I had everything I needed, I had enough of it, and I knew where it was. Now if I could only keep up that level of organization at home!"

Christopher Angell, the CEO and founder of GlucoLift glucose tablets, is a PWD and world traveler. Christopher shared one of his most amusing travel/airport security stories. *"I travel by air around 60 to 70 times a year, and the vast majority of those times without incident. I can count on my fingers the number of problems I've had with scanners/ pat-downs, metal detectors, or in-air concerns. Part of that comes from practice and preparation, but a lot of it is due to the fact that most of the time, people are reasonable and understanding. There are horror stories to be sure but, for every one of those, countless trips went smoothly.*

"Can you relate to my favorite travel story? I used to always keep my insulin pens in a Frio® case when I traveled. I was heading through security at San Diego's Lindbergh Field with a freshly plumped Frio® case in my carry-on. I did that all the time and never once had anyone comment on it. I never even bothered to take it out of my carry-on when I sent it through the X-ray. This time, I was stopped by an agent after going through the scanner.

"Agent: 'Sir, is this your bag?' Me: 'Yes.' Agent: 'Do you have

anything sharp or dangerous in it?' Me: 'A few syringes, but they have caps on them.' Agent: 'OK. Umm ... sir ... do you have ... do you have a burrito in your bag?'

    "*When he asked that, three things immediately popped into my head:*

    1. *I was in San Diego. Shouldn't they know what a burrito looks like?*

    2. *Since when are we not allowed to bring burritos on planes?*

    3. *I really wanted a burrito.*

Someday, I'd really like to see a burrito and a Frio® side-by-side on an X-ray machine."

For those of you who have never used one, Frio® cases are sleeves of varying sizes and shapes that contain crystals that, when soaked in water for a few minutes, expand into a polymer gel. It has an outer layer made out of a wicking fabric that allows water to slowly evaporate, keeping the contents inside the sleeve at a constantly cool temperature. They look similar to small inflatable rafts. Christopher Angell says they are invaluable for those times when he knows he's going somewhere really hot and will be exposed to that heat for a long time.

Sean Busby is a professional snowboarder and Olympian as well as a person with type 1 diabetes. Sean is the founder of Riding on Insulin, a snowboarding camp for children with type 1 diabetes. He often snowboards in backcountry wilderness on expeditions. The expeditions last from hours to several days. Sean is planning to snowboard on his seventh continent. Through his travels, he has become a true expert in diabetes planning and organization.

"Anything can happen when you are snowboarding on an expedition in the wilderness. Before you leave for your trip, I strongly suggest you contact your insulin pump company. They usually have prototypes to take with you in case of a malfunctioning pump or supply problem. There is so much that can (and often does) go wrong when traveling. Being organized with your diabetes supplies and prepared with detailed information (about anything and everything) can reduce many potential problems."

Sean is also out of the country on snowboarding expeditions for a good percentage of the year. Since he chases winter, he is often crossing several time zones in a fairly short period of time. He says planning ahead is key!

"If I am going to Australia, for example, I start to adjust my pump weeks in advance so I'm prepared and organized for the time zone change. That way when I arrive in the country I'm able to take advantage of my time there rather than worrying too much about pump adjustment. I always discuss where I'm going and about how long I plan to travel with my doctor weeks before I leave. Together we plan on how to organize my supplies and how to adjust my pump."

Country music superstar and JDRF spokesperson **George Canyon** is a person with type 1 diabetes. George told us how preparing for a tour used to be a bit of a nightmare.

"When I get ready to go on the road, I try to keep my diabetes supplies, medications, and insulin well organized. But I remember way back (almost 25 years ago) when I went into the music business professionally, going on the road was quite a challenge! I always tried to figure out how many vials of insulin I was going to need, how many needles I was going to need, how many test strips, and all that stuff. Nowadays, being on an Animas Insulin Pump makes life really, really simple. Now I make sure to have a 'diabetes supply pack' always ready. I plan to stay organized and have improved my diabetes management while I'm on the road."

Travel Checklists

Here's a quick list of items to have written and with you at all times:
- ☐ Medications (include dosage)
- ☐ Vitamins and supplements
- ☐ Pharmacy contact information for both home and away
- ☐ Doctors' contact information
- ☐ Emergency contact numbers
- ☐ Local grocery or convenience stores' phone numbers and hours of operation

Apps for Travel

Topic	iPhone	Android
Doctor Appointments	ZocDoc	ZocDoc
Time Zones	Clock	World Clock & Widget
Drug Stores	CVS, Walgreens, RiteAid	CVS, Walgreens, RiteAid
EHR	MyChart, iBlueButton, Kaiser Permanente, DrChrono	MyChart, iBlueButton, Kaiser Permanente, DrChrono EHR, Medilog: My Family EMR Diary, Health Tracker Free
Log Blood Sugar	Gucomo, Glucose Buddy, Vree, iBGStar glucose meter	Glucose Buddy, Glucool Diabetes Premium
Nutrition	Carb Counting with Lenny, Diabetes Nutrition by Fooducate, diabetes IQ, Eat Smart with Hope Warshaw, My Net Diary	Carb Counting with Lenny, Fooducate, Eat Smart with Hope Warshaw, My Net Diary, OnTrack Diabetes, Calorie Counter Pro
Insurance	Aetna Mobile, My Humana Mobile, Blue Finder	Aetna Mobile, My Humana Mobile, Blue Finder
Weather	Weather, The Weather Channel, MyRadar	The Weather Channel
Grocery	Shopper, Grocery IQ, Grocery Smarts Coupon Shopper	Shopper, Grocery IQ, Grocery Smarts Coupon Shopper
Portions	Figwee	Carbs and Cals
Water Tracker	8 Glasses a Day, Water Me, Water Tracker, Water Logged	Water Bot, Hydrator, Tracker Savvy Water Log Widget
Alerts	Clock, App reSolutions, My 'LilCoach, Eat Better Goal Getter	Eat Better Goal Getter
Taxi	Uber (private car), Taxi, Taxi Magic	Uber (private car), Taxi Magic

Source: Adapted from *An App A Day* and *An App A Day for Health Professionals*, © 2012, Frederico Arts LLC; www.AppyLiving.com.

Have a Backup Plan

Send copies of important information and your detailed itinerary to a family member, neighbor, or assistant. Make your travel stress free!

We know that in this day and age it is easier to keep all your information on one of your many electronic devices, and there are plenty of cool apps that can replace all those paper printouts. However, try not to rely solely on electronics. Lost chargers, dead batteries, or limited cell or web service can leave you stranded. Keep an electronic and hard copy version of all your critical information on hand.

> If you plan to travel abroad, have all your medical information converted to the language of the country you are planning to visit. Carry this information with you at all times.

Supplies

☐ Always carry at least double the amount of your medications, including insulin and diabetes supplies. What if you wind up

> Create one sheet with all your important information. Convert it to a PDF and save it in a Dropbox or Evernote folder that you can access from anywhere. Or, snap a photo with your phone for a quick reference.

staying longer than you had planned? Bad weather or airport delays can extend your trip. So don't skimp on extra supplies.

☐ Keep your supplies within reach. Don't store supplies in an overhead airplane bin that you can't get to during a bumpy flight.

☐ Clearly mark all your diabetes supplies and include the pharmacy's original labeling when possible.

> Keep all your supplements and medications organized with a pill organizer. We like the one from Lewis N. Clark (www.amazon.com). With removable see-through pouches for day and night and slide-lock closures, you'll never miss a dosage.

Snacks

☐ Pack nonperishable snacks. Bring sports bars or a homemade trail mix of nuts and dried fruit. If your travel is delayed, test your blood sugar and eat a snack as necessary. Your snacks can help you prevent or treat a low blood sugar. Glucose tablets or gels or another fast-acting source of carbohydrate are a must when you travel.

☐ Bring extra foil, clear wrap, and storage bags. These items may come in handy when you pack snacks for your return trip. Do you usually use measuring spoons or cups? If it will make you feel more confident about your portion control, bring along a few measuring supplies.

☐ Call the hotel ahead of time to request a refrigerator for your room. You can ask the hotel to empty the minibar before you check in so that you have ample room for your refrigerated supplies and snacks.

Dining Out

Do you find it difficult to eat out in restaurants when you travel? Portion sizes can be huge and may provide extra carb grams, calories, and a lot of excess sodium and fat. Take control of your food while eating out with these terrific tips:

- Check out the menu of the restaurant in advance so that you can make appropriate choices. Try to steer clear of all-you-can-eat buffets. Many hotel concierges keep restaurant menus on hand, so enlist their help.
- Look for key healthy words on menus, such as broiled, roasted, or grilled.

Use a hanging toiletry bag as a nonperishable snack and supply carrier. Find one that has elastic bands and zippered compartments. Once you arrive at your destination, just open the bag and hang for easy access. Now your snacks will be contained and easily accessible.

- Ask for food to be prepared with less salt and order all dressings and sauces on the side. To avoid blood sugar spikes, find out what's in the sauce on your food as well.
- Be vocal. Do you have a specific food allergy or intolerance? Or, do they not have on the menu what you would like? If you don't see what you want, ask for it anyway. Don't be afraid to ask for healthy substitutions. Many restaurants will accommodate your requests. You aren't the first to ask and you won't be the last.
- If you are visiting a country whose residents speak a foreign language, learn a few important menu phrases in that language. Better to be prepared so you can order stress free.
- Avoid portion distortion. Choose the smallest meal size. For example, order a lunch-sized entrée or appetizer for dinner or, if dining out with a friend, split an entrée. Consider sharing a dessert or ordering a "kiddie-size" portion.
- Eliminate temptation! When you order, ask for half the meal to be placed in a doggie-bag before it reaches your table.
- Stand strong when you order. Try not to let your dining partner sabotage your healthy food choices. You can do it!
- Have a game plan. Try to eat at about the same time as you would if you were home. You will be more likely to manage your blood sugars if you eat your meals and test your blood sugars at the same time at or away from your home.
- If you plan to eat later than usual, make sure that you eat an additional snack prior to your meal. Bring a snack with you in

case your meal is delayed. You may also have to adjust your insulin or medications if you plan to eat much later than usual. Make sure you plan for slow service and adjust your insulin or medication accordingly.

George Canyon uses a travel case to keep him organized. George says, "*I've got my blue Camp Seale Harris (given to me as a gift when I talked with and performed for the kids at camp) to carry my insulin. I put everything in this bag. I carry all my meter information, my testing supplies, batteries, insulin, and reservoir systems in my cool Camp Seale Harris bag. I carry a few extra insulin needles, just in case, as well as an extra pump. Usually, it takes me about an hour to get all of that ready before I head out on the road. I always pack the night before, so I don't feel rushed in the morning.*"

Benno Schmidt III is a seasoned TV news reporter and TV host who has traveled the world. He is a person with type 1 diabetes and wears an insulin pump and CGM. We asked Benno about his routine. "*I strongly suggest bringing along extra supplies and prescriptions when traveling. I always keep extra tubing and a fresh reservoir in all of my travel bags. I also use my Test Meter Bag as my wallet. Although I carry it around like 'a man purse,' it holds all my necessary papers including my driver's license and important papers. That may sound strange, but I think it helps me stay organized and it's one less thing to carry.*"

Benno also reminded us that "diabetes supplies" doesn't just mean insulin, alcohol pads, syringes, and other specialized items. "*I need fresh AAA batteries first and foremost for my pump. My pump seems to eat them up! I learned this the hard way when I was reporting in Haiti and the Middle East. Would you believe that many folks actually and actively sell counterfeit batteries in many countries? No batteries, no pump, no insulin ... not good. Not good at all. So I bring at least 20 extra AAA batteries with me when traveling. I also try to find out in advance where I can purchase additional fresh batteries if necessary.*"

And **Sean Busby** told us that despite your best efforts at planning ahead, things sometimes don't go as planned. "*I know that fish contains healthy omega 3s, but the truth is that I don't eat any seafood! I was on an expedition to Iceland, where everyone caught his or her fish for practically every meal. I thought I was prepared by bringing along honey and beef jerky. But it didn't pass through customs! I had over $100 worth of food confiscated and thrown away. Since that time, I always check what's allowed through customs in the country that I'm visiting. It helps me organize my snacks and pack plenty of nonperishable items that I can turn to if I won't eat the food typical to the country I'm visiting.*"

Staying Healthy While on the Road

Follow these simple rules for optimum health while on the road!

Move. Plan to walk around a bit every hour when you travel by air, bus, train, or car. If you walk, you may help to prevent blood clots from forming. Need another reason to walk? You might be able to prevent blood clots *and* help to keep your blood sugars within range. Try to keep up with your exercise routine when away from home. Call ahead to find out if there is a gym or a walking path at your hotel. (Check out our chapter on exercise for more great ideas on how to stay active.)

Drink. Put yourself on a water schedule in order to stay hydrated. Although you might not feel thirsty, it's important to drink plenty of water. Look at your agenda for the day to plan to "fit your water in." Keep water handy in your car. Treat yourself to a bottle of water once you pass airport security. Need a reminder to drink plenty of water when you travel? Try one of these terrific apps— 8 Glasses a Day, Water Me, Water Tracker, Water Logged.

Snack. Take portioned snacks with you. If you travel by car, pack a cooler with some fruit, Greek yogurt, and a sandwich of lean turkey on whole grain bread. Keep some unsalted nuts, veggies, and hummus close by for a yummy snack. Take along a sandwich (such as turkey breast with low-fat Swiss cheese on whole grain bread) and some fruit on the plane.

Proximity. We've said it before, but it bears repeating—keep your must have diabetes travel supplies with you at all times. If you are planning

> Freeze water bottles the night before you leave. If you plan to travel by car, train, or bus, a frozen water bottle will help keep perishables cold and give you ample liquids while traveling.

225

to fly, keep your necessary supplies in your carry-on luggage. Even if your checked luggage is lost by the airline, you'll have your diabetes supplies with you. If you plan to travel by car, bus, or train, keep your diabetes supplies within reach. That way, your supplies will be kept in a temperature-controlled environment and close by in case you need anything.

Carry. Use a fanny pouch or small knapsack when you take a day trip. If you are away from your hotel or rental home for the day,

Benno Schmitt shares a story about a diabetes travel glitch. *"One time I lost my pump on a plane. As if traveling is not draining and tiring enough, I actually lost my pump. I got up to go to the bathroom and unplugged it, leaving it on my seat, hidden in the seat cushion. When I fly, my blood sugar tends to go low. My endocrinologist at the Diabetes Research Institute (DRI), Bresta Miranda-Palma, MD, has begged me repeatedly to use the bolus wizard. I have ADHD (attention deficit hyperactivity disorder) and often require immediate gratification with almost everything I do. So I wind up testing my blood sugars over and over again and taking tiny boluses of insulin to correct. Maybe I need to start to consider the bolus wizard. When I got off the plane, I hopped into a cab and drove to the nearest pharmacy. I had a prescription for Humalog insulin, which I injected immediately."* Over the past few weeks, Benno has started to use a CGM! He told us that he is now more confident about traveling and has had better control of his blood sugars while traveling through time zones. Good for you, Benno!

Use a WatchMinder (www.watchminder.com) to remind yourself to monitor your blood sugar levels or take your meds. A WatchMinder is a vibrating watch and reminder system that can be programmed to send you discreet alerts. Choose from over 65 preprogrammed reminder messages and then either set a fixed time or a time interval to cue you with your message. Never miss a blood sugar check again! Or, you can try one of the following time-alert apps—Clock, resolutions, MyLil'Coach, or Goal Getter.

load your knapsack with snacks, bottled water, your medical information, and daily diabetes supplies. No panic necessary if you decide to extend your day!

Disclosure. You can wear a fashionable medical ID bracelet or necklace. If you plan to travel with a friend or companion, please let them know that you have diabetes. Discuss the signs of hypoglycemia and show them where you keep your glucose tablets or fast-acting source of carbohydrate.

Checking Blood Sugar with ADHD—Remembering to Remember

Do you or someone you know have ADHD and diabetes? You might find it difficult to remember the multitude of tasks needed to plan and coordinate your travels and manage your diabetes at the same time. But as you know, it is crucial to test your blood sugar and eat properly when on the go. Please don't worry! We are here to help. Here are a few tips to help you if you have ADHD and diabetes:

- Set reminders and alerts on your phone at the beginning of each day to ensure you never forget to check your blood sugar and to eat your meals and snacks.
- Two heads are always better than one. Inform your travel companions or guides about your blood sugar testing schedule. If you lose track of time, someone can remind you.
- Place a rubberband or string around your finger or wrist as a visual cue.

George Canyon performs his music around the world. He also uses an insulin pump. We asked him how his insulin pump helps him when he travels and performs. "*How I use my pump often depends on the number of sets I'm performing as well as the length of my show. If I am doing a 90-minute show, sometimes I'll stay connected to my pump, depending on my blood sugars. Quite often I try to go onstage with a slightly higher blood sugar, just to make sure I don't go low. I have had incidents where I went low before. If I'm doing two 45-minute sets, which often we do in theatres, I'll actually disconnect my pump and on the break I'll put my pump back on. Other times I simply bolus as needed, and then return to the stage with the pump off. It just really depends on the show. That's the wonderful thing with my Animas Pump. The pump gives me freedom to choose what is best for me for many different situations. If I was still using injections, I would've probably had to endure many hypo- and hyperglycemic situations while onstage. For 22 years before the pump, I had to manage highs and lows by taking as many as* five shots of insulin every day! The pump has made traveling with diabetes much easier to manage. The pump has really given me so much more freedom! All of a sudden, it was like becoming 13 again (I was diagnosed at the age of 14). The pump makes my life so much easier."

We asked George how the pump has affected how he eats when he travels. "I've been to Afghanistan around six times. It's often difficult to schedule meals and choose healthy foods. I'm often on the run, and although I try to eat healthy and well-balanced meals, sometimes I just grab a few bites of food here and there. The pump is a great tool that usually helps me keep my blood sugars in range, even when I don't eat my typical diet. The great thing about using my pump when performing on the road is I can eat at various times. For example, if I come off a show and it's eleven o'clock at night, and I want to eat my supper then—that's when I eat my supper. It just makes it that much simpler."

George is committed to staying organized and sharing a positive message. "You can help to manage your diabetes if you stay organized. I tell kids all across North America to stay focused. Stay on a 'positive' road and do your best to manage your diabetes. Keep going forward on that right path. You might even fall off that path many, many times. Sometimes you might wake up in the morning with an elevated blood sugar. You might not even know why your blood sugar is high. We don't always know what causes our blood sugars to go high or low. Endocrinologists don't know why. Nobody knows why. Try not to get overwhelmed. Stay positive! I'm right here with you!"

Chapter Twelve

Tackling the Holiday Madness

HAVE YOU EVER FELT FRAZZLED AND SCATTERED during the holiday season? You're not alone. From Halloween to New Year's Day, we seem to have endless to-do lists added to our typical daily activities. You probably want to buy gifts for loved ones and friends and attend some holiday parties, too. However, we all know that many of these parties have a seemingly endless abundance of foods that are high in calories, salt, carbohydrates, and fat. Naturally, you want to feel your best during this jam-packed season. So remember to always try and do your best to properly manage your diabetes. You shouldn't expect to be perfect. But if you can keep your blood sugar in your target range, chances are you will be more likely to feel your best all season long.

How can you handle the additional festivities associated with this busy time of year and still stay organized? With some simple suggestions and organizing techniques, you can continue to successfully manage your diabetes throughout the holiday season. So please don't worry, we have some suggestions that will help you stay on track.

Keep to a Schedule

You've done an amazing job of organizing your morning, afternoon, and evening routines for most of the calendar year. But even we have to admit that it is an even bigger challenge to stick to your usual schedule during the holidays. Trust us—you *can* continue to test your blood sugar and (for the most part) eat nutritious and well-balanced meals during the holidays. Do your best to stick to your exercise and medication schedule, so that you are able to handle what many folks consider "the

Ginger Vieira is a PWD, author, and certified cognitive coach. *"When it comes to holiday foods and events, you can never test your blood sugar too often! If you're dosing insulin and constantly trying to estimate the carbohydrate quantities in certain foods, it's okay if you aren't the perfect carbohydrate-guessing robot. But always test your blood sugar more often in the hours after your holiday meal. Your extra effort can help make up for any inaccuracy in your estimation. Test, test, test!."*

Jim Turner, comedian, says, *"I always make the time to test! Nothing is more important. Not even holiday shopping. I have a jacket made by Scottevest that has like a hundred pockets. I carry my kit, glucose tabs, and granola bars with me all the time. I have also come around to the wonder of the continuous glucose monitor (CGM). It's my new best friend. I look at it constantly. I'm like a teenager checking his text messages constantly."* We can clearly picture Jim checking his CGM. If Jim can check, so can you!

most wonderful time of the year." Sometimes the holidays may include some additional pressures for you if you have diabetes and those may not always be so wonderful.

Have you ever had a low blood sugar episode during a shopping trip in an overcrowded mall during the month of December? If that's happened to you, chances are that you've vowed never to experience that uncomfortable and scary moment again. So, before you venture out for the day, plan to eat at (or as close as possible to) your usual mealtime.

Bring food with you, or check out the choices at the food court online before you leave the house. If you shop at a mall or walk from store to store, you might be adding a lot of mileage to your day. Make sure to keep an eye out for potential low blood sugar reactions.

Be Aware of BLTs—Bites, Licks, and Tastes

Have you ever noticed that there is an abundance of food everywhere you turn during the holiday season? Holiday cookie exchanges, office parties, Sunday brunch get-togethers, and the list goes on and on. You might be tempted to just try one bite of cake or one piece of candy. Remember that these bites, licks, and tastes can lead to an expanded waistline and an unusual rise in your blood sugar level. So, be aware as you navigate through the food maze during this busy time of year.

Ready to shop for the holidays? Make sure to bring along glucose tablets or some other fast-acting source of carbohydrate (such as a juice box or Skittles). Keep a few glucose tablets in your pocket or purse. If you plan to drive to your shopping destination, keep snacks and glucose tablets in the car. Your shopping trip may take longer than expected or you may get stuck in a traffic jam. Don't let a low blood sugar slow you down at the mall or on the drive home!

Eat What You Enjoy, But Watch Your Portions!

Do you have a special dish that you simply love to eat on Thanksgiving? Perhaps you salivate at the thought of biting into Aunt Edith's double-stuffed potatoes or your mom's pecan pie. Of course you can enjoy a few of your favorites, but watch your portions! Try to be proactive. For example, if the holiday meal is at a friend or relative's home, ask about the menu before you arrive.

Don't be shy! Ask your host any questions you may have about the menu. Chances are that your host will be accommodating and more than happy to tell you what's on the menu. He or she might even share a few secret recipe ingredients! Review the menu and select some of your favorites. Plan to have a small portion of a few special dishes. After all, you probably looked forward to this meal for the past several months, or maybe even since last year! Eat what you like, but try not to get carried away. And remember to test your blood sugar level regularly. Treat highs or lows as necessary. If you manage your diabetes well during the holidays, you can actually have your holiday cake and eat it, too.

How does Jim Turner stay active during the holidays? *"Staying physically active during the holidays is difficult because the school gymnasiums where I play my weekly basketball games are closed for a month. Fortunately, I have a dog! He needs to be walked daily. During the holidays, I make our walks longer. Getting my exercise during the holidays is one of those times of year that I have to work and plan extra hard to make sure I get my minutes in. I don't like to, but sometimes I'll actually keep a chart (ack!). My dog, Bob, makes the whole process easier because he gives me the woeful evil-eye whenever he feels neglected."*

Stay Physically Active

Do you usually go to the gym to work out? Chances are that during the holidays, you might not be able to get to the gym as regularly, but you should continue to be physically active. Exercise tends to reduce stress, burns calories, and may help to control your blood sugar levels. Would you like to start a new exercise tradition? During a holiday gathering (for example, Thanksgiving), play an active game of football outside. Try to sign up for a local "Turkey Trot" walk or run in your neighborhood. You'll feel energized before the holiday begins.

Monitor Your Alcohol Consumption

Have you ever felt stressed-out when you arrive at a holiday party, family gathering, or event? Do you immediately reach for an alcoholic beverage? Remember that if you have not yet eaten, an alcoholic beverage can pack a big punch and in some instances may significantly lower your blood sugar. So, start off with a diet soda or glass of sparkling water. If you drink too much alcohol, you might also lower your resolve to monitor what you eat. You might eat more unhealthy foods when you drink alcohol.

Drink Plenty of Water

Drink plenty of water to keep yourself well hydrated. Don't forget to drink plenty of fluids when the weather turns frosty or when you are extremely busy or stressed out.

Take a liquid measuring cup and a wine glass out of your cabinet at home. Measure out five ounces of water (which is the recommended serving of wine) and pour it into the wine glass. Now you will have a visual awareness of what a serving of wine is supposed to look like. Remember, you can decide when to say "stop" if a friend or relative is pouring a glass of wine for you at Christmas dinner.

Please don't rely on thirst to tell you to drink water! By the time you're thirsty, you might already be slightly dehydrated.

Don't Go into a Holiday Meal Hungry

Don't try to starve yourself earlier in the day or bank your calories in anticipation of the holiday meal. When you arrive at a party really hungry, you tend to devour appetizers and unhealthy carb-laden chips and dips. Therefore, you should try to have your usual healthy breakfast on the day of a holiday meal (and lunch if your meal is being served late in the day). If you have good blood sugar control as the holiday meal approaches, you'll be able to think clearly. *You* will be in control of your thoughts and of your food choices! You can have what you want, as long as you continue to monitor your blood sugar and try not to go completely overboard.

> Add a slice of lemon, lime, or cucumber to your water to make it even more tasty and delicious. Try some sparkling water instead of champagne. It looks festive and can be substituted for extra glasses of alcohol.

Keep Your Focus on Family and Friends

Celebrate the meaning of the holiday with the people you love, not just the food. Have you been harassed by a relative or friend who acts like "the diabetes food monitor" at a holiday gathering? These are folks who feel the need to comment or question your food choices. Uncle Marvin might blurt out, "You're a diabetic. You shouldn't be eating that!" Aunt

When going to a party, offer to bring a nutritious dish that you enjoy. How about a veggie platter with homemade salsa or hummus, or a tray of roasted asparagus? For dessert, offer to bring a seasonal fresh fruit platter topped with a dollop of Greek yogurt, slivered almonds, and a dash of cinnamon. Your host will appreciate your generosity, and you'll have a guaranteed healthy choice at the holiday meal.

Matilda might announce that she also has diabetes and her doctor told her to only eat dry white meat turkey and plain green beans over the holiday. She might even make this ridiculous statement while glaring in your direction. Your response to any of these silly questions or comments can be a simple, "I've got it under control." Because you do! And then you can change the subject to a hot-button topic such as politics or religion. What a way to successfully switch subjects and start a lively (and possibly memorable) discussion.

Organizing Tips for Stress-Free Holidays

The holidays can be hectic and overwhelming at times. However, if you manage your activities and plan your time properly, you can have an enjoyable and less stressful holiday season. Plus, you can keep your blood sugars in control at the same time. We have you covered with these tips on how to get and stay organized!

Make a master holiday to-do list. Create a list of everything you need to do and want to get done for the holidays. Whether you write your task list in a notebook, on your smartphone, or a bulletin board in your office, make sure your list is in one place and easily accessible. Doing a brain dump will take the remembering out of remembering and you'll feel in control in an instant. Just remember to use whatever system works best for you.

Use a calendar to create deadlines. Once you have your main list of to-dos, break them into smaller tasks and place deadlines for each on your calendar. For example, if you like to send out holiday cards, your list might look something like this: Schedule date to take family photograph; create card on publishing site; update mailing list; stuff, stamp, and address envelopes; drop envelopes

Jim Turner says *"I've been very lucky. My family and most of my friends know not to be poking their nose where it doesn't belong. However, there is the occasional nosy poker in the world of food police—and diabetes police and other cultural police. My response is always the same. I listen politely and I say, 'Thank you so much. I appreciate that. I hadn't thought of that. I'll try it your way. Thank you.' Then I change the conversation. If the conversation persists, I politely—and quickly—change company."*

off at post office. Try to follow a step-by-step plan to reduce your stress and achieve your goals. Make sure to give yourself ample time to accomplish most of what's on your list.

Plan ahead. Shop for gifts in June. Wrap presents in September. Cook and freeze (and don't forget to label) in November. There are endless tasks that can be done ahead of time. Try not to save everything for the last minute. Plan ahead so you will enjoy the holiday to the fullest!

Write down everything in a paper calendar (or on your phone) to help keep track of appointments and events. You can even schedule your workouts after you throw in a load of laundry. Make appointments with yourself. This will give you peace of mind during this busy time of year!

Clear the clutter. The key to a peaceful, relaxed, and comfortable home during the holidays is a clutter-free environment. Whether it's purging the pantry or lightening up the linen closet, feeling organized will help you reduce your stress. Extra bonus? By decluttering your home *before* the holidays, you will make added room for any gifts you receive.

Organize your shopping trips. No one wants to make endless trips to the stores during the holiday. Try to organize your to-dos by store and you will save time, money, and gas. Or, better yet, shop online!

Think clutter-free gift giving. Does your babysitter really need another candle? Does your child's teacher need more stationery? We're thinking no. Movie passes, restaurant vouchers, cooking classes, even museum memberships are clever and clutter-free gifts that say "enjoy an experience." So, gift your friends and family with consumable gifts and bring the holiday spirit home. Bonus? You can store these cards or certificates in one convenient place before the holiday.

Ask for help. We're going to say it again. Ask for help. Don't think you can do it all, because you can't. Trust us. We've been there. If your sister-in-law offers to bring the salad, say yes. If you need help in the kitchen while preparing the holiday dinner, recruit your guests to join you to peel potatoes or have someone set the table. They will feel so appreciative that you asked.

Take care of yourself. During the holidays, we are all consumed with checking things off our ever growing to-do list. Well, please remember to put "you" on that list! You still need to manage your diabetes during this busy time of year. Take an exercise class or a walk with a friend. Take a quick retreat into a quiet space and take a few deep breaths. Do anything that will rejuvenate you and reset your mind and spirit.

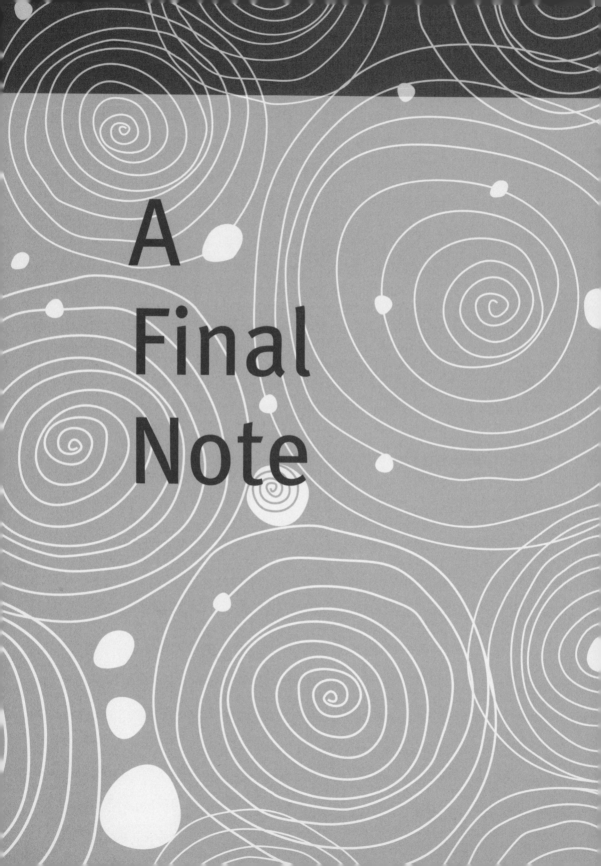

A
Final
Note

YOU DID IT! You're now on your way to a more organized and better managed diabetes life. Remember, your daily diabetes management requires a plan each and every day. And permanent lifestyle changes take time. Anyone can try a quick fix. But we want you to be successful with healthy changes that last a lifetime. Long-term organizational change requires figuring out what works for YOU and your life. After reading this book, we hope that incorporating one positive organizational change will lead to another. And once you've organized one area of your life, you are inspired to start on another.

We also hope that by following our suggestions, even if it's only a few of them, you may start to see some overall improvements in your health. Now you can see how staying organized may help you manage your diabetes and overall health. Notice also that all of these positive effects can multiply because, once you start to feel better, you'll want to continue doing what you did to get you there.

We've obviously given you oodles of information. We don't expect you to absorb everything in one shot and immediately start a brand new routine. We suggest you start by creating a short list of basic goals and then adopting a few suggestions and guidelines to support them. Once you've incorporated those changes in your life and are comfortable with them, you can move on to add a few more of our strategies and routines. Just remember to go at your own pace.

And now that you've finished the book, please don't let it just gather dust on your bookshelf. We've designed the book to be a valuable resource you can refer to over and over again, and hopefully find something new and useful each time you do. So, go back from time to time and open it up. Perhaps you'll find a few more tips and tools that you weren't ready for the first time you read it. Or you might feel inspired to read it all the way through again for a quick refresher. Either way, give yourself credit for your accomplishments. We are thrilled to be part of your journey.

Wishing you good health and organizing success ...

Acknowledgments

We would like to thank the following incredibly knowledgeable and talented professionals for their guidance, contributions, advice, and encouragement: Stephanie Brenner, MS, RD; R. Keith Campbell, PharmD, MBA, CDE, FAADE; Vincent Carvelli; Diane de Jesús, RD; Alyssa De Monte; Monica Dennis; Nicola Farman; Paula Ford-Martin; Riva Greenberg; Deborah Hoffman; Rebecca Kaye, RD; and Tracy Stopler, MS, RD. Thank you for making this book a reality.

Contributors

Thank you to all who shared advice, stories, and encouragement.

Beverly Adler, PhD, CDE
Christopher Angell
Jason Baker, MD
Sean Busby
George Canyon
Tony Cervati
Carrie Cheadle, MA
Matt Corcoran, MD, CDE
Will Cross
Catherine Frederico, MS, RD, LDN
Scott Herman
Jeff Hitchcock
Mary Ann Hodorowicz, RD, LDN, MBA, CDE, CEC
Tom and Jill Karlya
Francine Kaufman, MD
Robert Lewis

Annette and Ryan Maloney
Robert Oringer and Family
Robin Plotkin, RD, LDN
Kyrra Richards
Gary Scheiner, MS, CDE
Benno Schmidt III
Toby Smithson, RDN, LDN, CDE
Phil and Joanna Southerland
Kerri Sparling
Howard Steinberg
Nat Strand, MD
Max Szadek
Sam Talbot
Jim Turner
Ginger Vieira
Saul Zuckman

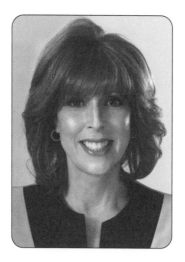

SUSAN WEINER, MS, RDN, CDE, CDN, is a renowned diabetes educator and lecturer who earned a Master's Degree in Applied Physiology and Nutrition from Columbia University and a Certificate of Training in Adult Weight Management from the Academy of Nutrition and Dietetics. She is a contributing medical producer for *dLife TV*, a member of dLife's medical advisory board, and the food and nutrition expert for dlife.com. Susan authors articles for Walgreens' *Diabetes and You* and has been the lead CDE for DiabetesSisters.org, an organization that supports women with diabetes.

From her active private practice in Long Island, New York, Susan helps individuals and families achieve their nutrition and health goals. She maintains a website at SusanWeinerNutrition.com and was recently voted one of the top 10 nutritionist bloggers for diabetes education by iVillage.

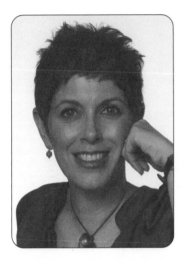

LESLIE JOSEL is an acclaimed authority on chronic disorganization and hoarding issues. She is a member of the National Association of Professional Organizers and has received its Golden Circle distinction. Leslie has also received ADHD and Hoarding Specialist certifications from the Institute for Challenging Disorganization. Her practice, Order Out of Chaos, provides professional organizing services to the chronically disorganized as well as individuals, families, and students needing help with time management and organization.

Leslie has appeared on TLC's hit television show *Hoarding: Buried Alive*, the Cooking Channel's special *Stuffed: Food Hoarders*, and *The Better Show* as an organizational expert. She is the creator of the award-winning *Academic Planner: A Tool for Time Management*. She speaks and teaches on organizational issues, special needs, and women's entrepreneurship.

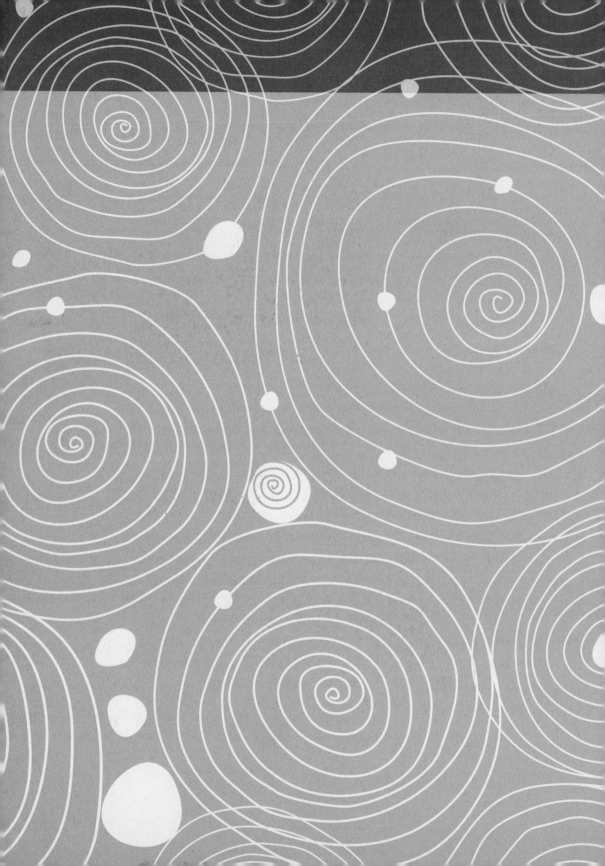